Doppler Ultrasound in Cardiology

Physical Principles and Clinical Applications

Doppler Ultrasound in Cardiology

Physical Principles and Clinical Applications

LIV HATLE, M.D.

Section of Cardiology
Regional Hospital
and
Department of Medicine
University of Trondheim
Trondheim, Norway

BJØRN ANGELSEN, DR. TECHN.

Associate Professor
Division of Engineering Cybernetics
The Norwegian Institute of Technology
and
Scientist
Automatic Control Division
The Foundation of Scientific and Industrial Research
The Norwegian Institute of Technology
Trondheim, Norway

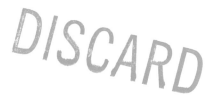

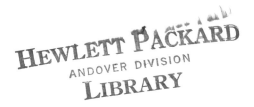

Lea & Febiger   1982   Philadelphia

Lea & Febiger
600 Washington Square
Philadelphia, PA 19106
U.S.A.

Library of Congress Cataloging in Publication Data

Hatle, Liv.
    Doppler ultrasound in cardiology.

    Contributors, Alf O. Brubakk, Svein E. Gisvold, Kjell Kristoffersen.
    Bibliography: p.
    Includes index.
    1. Ultrasonic cardiography. 2. Doppler effect.
I. Angelsen, Bjørn.   II. Title. [DNLM: 1. Ultrasonics—Diagnostic use. 2. Heart diseases—
Diagnosis. 3. Physics. WG 141.5E2 H361d]
    RC683.5.U5H37   1982   616.1'207543   82-9974
    ISBN 0-8121-0852-3   AACR2

PRINTED IN THE UNITED STATES OF AMERICA

Print No. 3 2 1

Preface

Recent years have shown much development in the application of ultrasonic techniques for noninvasive diagnosis of the cardiovascular system. The largest interest has been in ultrasonic imaging, using the amplitude of the backscattered ultrasound. The Doppler shift of the backscattered sound has been used to measure the velocity of blood flow. This has many interesting applications in the diagnosis and assessment of valve functioning and shunts. The information that is obtained by the Doppler techniques complements the information obtained by imaging. The usefulness of the technique has, however, been overshadowed by the almost explosive evolution in real-time two-dimensional imaging of the heart. In addition, it has not been clearly recognized that the Doppler signal itself is often a better guide than imaging for the localization of disturbed flow within the heart.

This occurs because the transducer directions that produce good image recordings usually do not produce the best Doppler recordings. Therefore, if one strains to obtain good images, the Doppler recording often suffers. Doppler measurements might also be somewhat more mysterious than imaging, since it seems easier to learn to relate to an image than to an obscure sound and a spectral tracing. This is probably caused by a lack of educational material. Once the basic principles of the technique are familiar, the ease of use is similar to that of imaging.

This book is intended as an introductory text to the use of ultrasonic Doppler techniques for cardiac diagnosis. Chapters 2 and 3 present the physics of blood flow and the principles of ultrasonic Doppler techniques. Chapters 4, 5, and 6 discuss clinical application in cardiac diagnosis. In Chapter 7, measurement of aortic flow velocity to obtain cardiac output is discussed, and Chapter 8 reviews methods of spectral analysis that are especially useful for Doppler signal analysis. This chapter is intended for readers with some technical background who are being introduced to the method.

Parts of Chapters 2 and 3 might be found somewhat technical. It is not necessary to grasp these chapters in full detail before reading the clinical portions of the book. The following introductory reading path is therefore suggested:

Chapter 1
Chapter 2, Section 2.1
Chapter 3, Sections 3.3 through 3.6
Chapters 4, 5, 6, and 7

The rest of Chapters 2 and 3 can then be read as needed.

All the clinical material presented in the book is obtained without the assistance of imaging. The combined use of Doppler measurements with 2D imaging could be useful. However, present combinations with 2D imaging have resulted in trade-offs in the sensitivity of the Doppler system which make them less suitable than a single Doppler system in many situations.

Trondheim, Norway   Liv Hatle

Trondheim, Norway   Bjørn Angelsen

Acknowledgments

The material presented in this book results from a seven-year combined technical and clinical program at the University of Trondheim, Norway, for the development of ultrasonic Doppler techniques for cardiovascular diagnosis. The work has been funded by grants from the University of Trondheim, The Royal Norwegian Council for Scientific and Industrial Research, The Norwegian Council on Cardiovascular Diseases, Forenede Liv Life Insurances, Forretningsbankens Fund for Bioengineering Research, Autronica A/S, Trondheim, and Vingmed A/S, Oslo.

Several persons have participated in the work. We especially wish to acknowledge K. Kristoffersen, M.Sc., who has written part of Chapter 6 and contributed to the essential parts of the instrumentation and measurements presented in this chapter. We also wish to thank him for his cooperation during the work as well as his suggestions and comments on the technical parts of the book. We want to offer a special thanks to R. Aaslid, Dr. Philos., and A.O. Brubakk, Dr. Med., for stimulating discussions and cooperation throughout the research. We also thank Professor J.G. Balchen, head of Division of Engineering Cybernetics, The Norwegian Institute of Technology, and Professor R. Rokseth, head of Section of Cardiology, University of Trondheim, for continuous encouragement and support throughout the work.

L.H.
B.A.

Contributors

ALF O. BRUBAKK, M.D.
Department of Clinical Physiology
University of Trondheim
Trondheim, Norway

SVEIN E. GISVOLD, M.D.
Department of Clinical Physiology
University of Trondheim
Trondheim, Norway

KJELL KRISTOFFERSEN, M.Sc.
Division of Engineering Cybernetics
Department of Electrical Engineering
Norwegian Institute of Technology
Trondheim, Norway

Contents

1

Introduction

1.1 THE DOPPLER EFFECT

If a person is moving *toward* a sound source, he will hear a tone with *higher* frequency than when he is at rest. If he is moving *away* from the source, he will hear a tone with *lower* frequency. The same is observed when the source is moving and the observer is at rest (Figure 1.1).

Christian Johann Doppler (1803-1853), an Austrian physicist, was the first to describe this effect. The change in frequency is called the *Doppler shift* in frequency, or simply the *Doppler frequency.*

The effect is found with all types of waves where the source and the receiver are moving relative to each other. In his paper of 1842, Doppler described how the color of the light from a star, in the same way as the pitch of a sound, is changed by the relative motion between source and observer. The same effect is used with radar waves to measure the speed of cars. When steering a boat against the waves, one will observe a higher frequency of the waves than when steering away from the waves. In everyday life one can observe the Doppler effect from a car siren or a train whistle. When an ambulance is approaching, for example, a higher pitch of the siren is heard than after it has passed. If the change in pitch is a whole tone step, the velocity of the car is approximately 70 km/h (45 mph).

1.2 CLINICAL USE OF ULTRASONIC DOPPLER TECHNIQUES

Ultrasound, like ordinary sound, is acoustic waves, but with a frequency above the audible range (20 to 20,000 Hz). For diagnostic purposes, frequencies in the range of 1 to 10 MHz* are used. At such high frequencies the sound tends to move along straight lines like a beam of light, and can be directed into the body from a handheld transducer.

The major application of diagnostic ultrasound has been for *imaging* of tissue structures. In these techniques the backscattered sound from tissue interfaces is used to generate an image as in radar and underwater sonar. The

*MHz = one million cycles per second

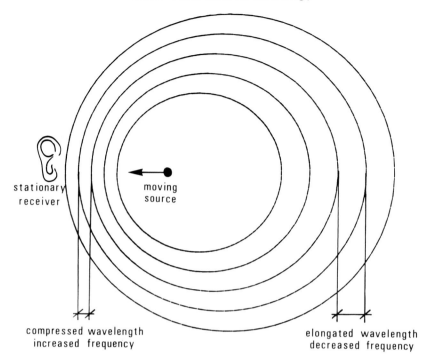

stationary
receiver

moving
source

compressed wavelength
increased frequency

elongated wavelength
decreased frequency

Fig. 1–1.   Illustration of the Doppler effect.

first use of the Doppler shift of ultrasound to measure the velocity of blood flow started at about the same time as ultrasonic imaging.[1-3] The earliest application was for qualitative evaluation of peripheral blood flow.[4,5] It has also been used together with an inflatable cuff to measure blood pressure,[6,7] and has been found especially valuable for measurement of blood pressure in the legs.[8] When it is used with a servo system for cuff inflation, it is even possible to obtain noninvasive recordings of pressure waveforms.[9] Light, et al. demonstrated the possibility of measuring the blood flow velocity in the aorta.[10]

For all these measurements a continuous wave instrument was used. Peronneau, et al.[11] and Baker[12] later introduced the pulsed ultrasonic Doppler instrument, by which the velocity in a small range cell can be studied. This makes it suitable for measurements in the heart, since velocities in the different cavities and valve areas can be studied selectively. Scanning the range cell along the ultrasonic beam allows velocity profiles to be obtained. Later on, pulsed instruments were developed that give a real-time presentation of time-variable velocity profiles.[13-15]

The main advantage of ultrasonic Doppler techniques is that measurements can be performed noninvasively.[16] Invasive measurements have been taken with Doppler transducers mounted at the tip of a catheter[17] and have been used in measurements of aortic, coronary, and intracardiac blood flow velocities.[18-21] In vascular surgery, measurements have been done directly on vessels.[22-29] This has an advantage over other methods, such as electromagnetic measurements, which require vessel dissection. It has also been used for guidance during vascular surgery in the brain.[30-32] In noninvasive measurements in the heart and larger vessels, an ultrasonic frequency of 1 to 3 MHz can be used. For invasive measurements and for noninvasive measurements in peripheral vessels, 5 to 10 MHz ultrasound has been used. Experiments with 20 MHz ultrasound have been performed.[33]

One disadvantage of the technique has been the problem of quantifying the results. This has probably been a hindrance for a wider clinical application of the method. Holen, et al. have published a method by which the pressure drop across a flow obstruction can be estimated.[34,35] The basis for this method is that an obstruction produces a marked increase in velocity, as shown for a mitral valve stenosis in Figure 1.2. The increase in velocity requires a pressure drop that can be obtained from the Bernoulli equation. The method provides valuable information complementary to imaging in the assessment of valvular obstructions and other lesions that produce high-velocity jets, such as valve regurgitations and ventricular septal defects.[36-40] The Doppler effect can also be used for accurate timing of valve opening and closure.[41]

The Doppler shift depends on the angle between the ultrasonic beam and the direction of the blood velocity. This angle is unknown in many situations.

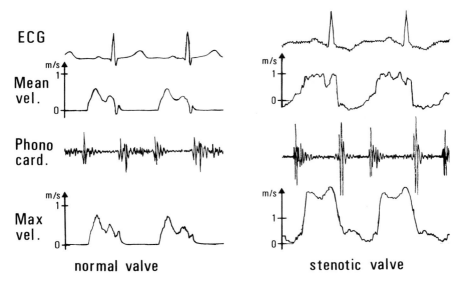

normal valve   **stenotic valve**

Fig. 1–2. **Blood velocity through a normal and a stenotic mitral valve. Note the increase in velocity in mitral stenosis.**

For measurements of blood velocity through the heart valves, it is often possible to place the transducer so that the angle is small and can be approximated to zero. This is necessary in order to quantify the results.

With ultrasonic Doppler methods, blood flow velocity and not volumetric flow rate is detected. The relationship between velocity and volumetric flow rate is discussed in Chapter 2. With a pulsed instrument, the maximum velocity that can be measured is limited because of a phenomenon called *frequency aliasing.* This introduces ambiguity in determining the velocity as discussed in Sections 3.3 and 3.6.

When the velocity limit is exceeded, as often occurs in various heart lesions, high Doppler shifts are mapped onto Doppler shifts with the opposite sign. This can indicate a false diagnosis of turbulence even if the flow is laminar. In the diagnosis of flow disturbances in the heart, turbulence has probably been emphasized too much, since even nonturbulent disturbed flow can have a turbulent appearance with existing pulsed instruments.

The continuous wave instrument does not have this aliasing limitation, and can therefore be used to record high velocities in the heart. The lack of range resolution does not usually create problems if one is interested in maximum velocities only. The high velocities can be localized using the pulsed technique. A combined instrument that can be switched between the pulsed and the continuous mode is, therefore, useful.

The signal processing used in earlier instruments (zero crossing detector,[42] Time Interval Histogram[43-45]) has limitations in producing adequate information about the blood flow velocity. *Spectral analysis* retrieves all information in the Doppler signal. A review of methods for spectral analysis is presented in Chapter 8. In our clinical work we have mainly used a simple maximum and mean frequency estimator which provides the main information in the signal found to be of clinical value (see Section 3.5). Spectral analysis is also shown to indicate how the single frequency estimators relate to the spectrum.

When *complex* spectral analysis is used, it is possible to extend the maximum velocity that can be measured with a pulsed instrument by a factor of two. This is discussed in Sections 3.6, 8.3, and 8.4C. In the case of a poor signal-to-noise ratio, it can also be advantageous to use full-spectrum analysis since the eye is a good detector for extracting the signal out from the noise. Figure 1.3 shows the Doppler unit with the spectrum analyzer.

M-mode has usually been used for guidance of the location of the range cell with pulsed instruments.[43] This has not been done in the work presented here for several reasons. Doppler measurements are performed with different transducer positions than for standard M-mode examination. For example, for measurements of mitral flow velocity, the beam is pointed from the apex of the heart so that it is in the direction of the flow. For M-mode measurements, the beam is pointed at right angles to the leaflets and the blood velocity direction. The requirements for optimizing the Doppler system are

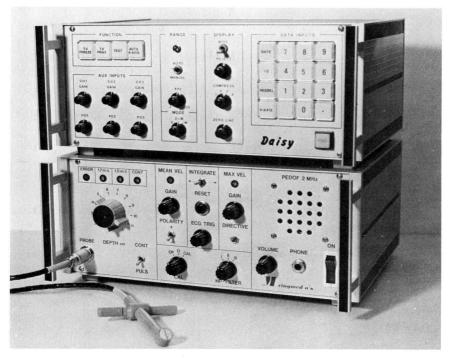

Fig. 1–3. Doppler unit and spectrum analyzer (Vingmed a/s, Oslo, Norway).

also different than the requirements for optimizing the M-mode system. Excluding the M-mode allows a more sensitive Doppler instrument to be designed. The range cell can also be localized within the heart using the Doppler signal only (see Chapter 4). Occasionally, it can even be easier to use the Doppler signal for localization than the M-mode, as for the aortic valve measured from the apex of the heart.

REFERENCES

1. Satumora S.: Ultrasonic Doppler method for the inspection of cardiac functions. J. Acoust. Soc. Am. 1957; 29:1181-1185.
2. Franklin D.L., Schlegal W.A., Rushmer R.F.: Blood flow measured by Doppler frequency shift of backscattered ultrasound. Science 1961; 134: 564-565.
3. Edler I., Lindstrøm K.: *In:* Ultrasonographic Medica. Vol. III. Edited by Bock J., Ossoing K., et al. Verlag Wiener Med. Akad. 1971; 455-461.
4. Fronek A., Johansen K.H., Dilley R.B.: Noninvasive physiologic tests in the diagnosis and characterization of peripheral occlusive disease. Am. J. Surg. 1973; 126: 205-214.
5. Blackshear W.M., Jr., Phillips D.J., Chibos P.M., Harley J.D., Thiele B.L., Strandness D.E., Jr. Carotid artery velocity patterns in normal and stenotic vessels. Stroke 1980; 11: 67-71.
6. Ware R.W.: New approaches to the indirect measure of human blood pressure. Third Nat. Biom. Sci. Instr. Symp., Instr. Soc. of Am., BM-65, Dallas 1965.

7. Alexander H., Cohen M.L., Steinfeld L.: Criteria in the choice of an occluding cuff for the indirect measurement of blood pressure. Med. Biol. Eng. Comput. 1977; 15: 2-10.
8. Yao J.S.T., Hobbs J.T., Irvine W.T.: Ankle systolic pressure measurements in arterial disease affecting the lower extremities. Br. J. Surg. 1969; 56: 676-679.
9. Aaslid R., Brubakk A.O.: Accuracy of an ultrasound Doppler servo method for noninvasive determination of instantaneous and mean arterial blood pressure. Circulation 1981; 64: 753-759.
10. Light L.H., Cross G.: Cardiovascular data by transcutaneous aorta velography. *In:* Blood Flow Measurement. Edited by Robert C. London, Sector Publishing Limited, 1972.
11. Peronneau P., Deloche A., Bui-Mong-Hung, Hinglais J.: Debitmetrie ultrasonore: Développements et application expérimentales. Europ. Surg. Res. 1969; 1: 147-156.
12. Baker D.W.: Pulsed ultrasonic Doppler blood-flow sensing. IEEE Trans. on S and US. 1970; SU-17: 170-185.
13. Peronneau P.A., Bugnon A., Bournat J.P., Xhaard M., Hinglais J.: Instantaneous bi-dimensional blood velocity profiles in the major vessels by a pulsed ultrasonic Doppler velocimeter. *In:* Ultrasonics in medicine. Edited by de Vlieger M., et al. Amsterdam, Excerpta Medica/American Elsevier, 1974; 259-266.
14. Granchamp P.A.: A novel pulsed directional Doppler velocimeter; The phase detection profilometer. *In:* Proceedings Second European Congress Ultrasonics in Medicine. Amsterdam, Excerpta Medica 1975; 137-143.
15. Brandestini M.: Topoflow—A digital full range Doppler velocity meter. IEEE Trans. on S and US 1978; SU-25: 287-293.
16. Mills C.J.: Measurements of pulsatile flow and flow velocity. *In:* Cardiovascular Dynamics. Edited by Bergel D.H. London, Academic Press, 1972; Vol. 1: 51-90.
17. Stegall H.F., Stone H.L., Bishop V.S., Laenger C.: A catheter-tip pressure and velocity sensor. Proc. 20th Am. Conf. Eng. Med. Biol. 1967; 27: 4.
18. Benchimol A., Desser K.B., Gartlan J.L.: Bidirectional blood flow velocity in the cardiac chambers and great vessels studied with the Doppler ultrasonic flowmeter. Am. J. Med. 1972; 52: 467-473.
19. Benchimol A., Desser K.B., Gartlan J.L.: Left ventricular blood flow velocity in man studied with the Doppler ultrasonic flowmeter. Am. Heart J. 1973; 85: 294-301.
20. Reid J.M., Davis D.L., Ricketts H.J., Spencer M.P.: A new Doppler flowmeter system and its operation with catheter mounted transducers. *In:* Cardiovascular Applications of Ultrasound. Edited by Reneman R.S. New York, Elsevier North-Holland 1974; 108-124.
21. Benchimol A., Stegall H.F., Gartlan J.L.: A new method to measure phasic coronary blood velocity in man. Am. Heart J. 1971; 81: 93-101.
22. Vatner S.F., Franlin D., van Clitters R.L.: Simultaneous comparison and calibration of the Doppler and electromagnetic flow meters. J. Appl. Physiol. 1970; 29: 907-910.
23. Reneman R.S., Clarke H.F., Simmons N., Spencer M.P.: In vitro comparison of electromagnetic and Doppler flowmeters. Physiologist 1971; 14: 218.
24. Lo Gerfo F.W., Corson J.D.: Quantitative ultrasonic blood flow measurements in Dacron grafts. Surgery 1976; 79: 569-572.
25. Myhre H.O., Krose A.J.: Ultrasound in the study of peripheral blood circulation. Acta Chir. Scand. 1979; Suppl. 488: 56-61.
26. FitzGerald D.E., Fortescue-Webb C.M., Ekestrøm S., Liljeqvist L., Nordhus O.: Monitoring coronary artery blood flow by Doppler shift ultrasound. Scand. J. Thorac. Cardiovasc. Surg. 1977; 11: 119-123.
27. Moulder P.V., Teague M., Manuele V.J., Brunswick R.A., Daicoff G.R.: Intraoperative Doppler coronary artery finder. Ann. Thorac. Surg. 1977; 24: 430-432.
28. Wright C., Doty D., Eastham C., Laughlin D., Krumm P., Mareus M.: A method for assessing the physiological significance of coronary obstructions in man at cardiac surgery. Circulation 1980; 62: I 111-I 115.
29. Brooks J.D., Magrath R.A., Beauchamp R.A., Clark R.E.: Determination of coronary blood flow following coronary artery bypass surgery using a bidirectional Doppler system: An alternative. J. Extra-Corp. Techn. 1980; 12: 89-94.
30. Nornes H., Grip A., Wikeby P.: Intraoperative evaluation of cerebral hemodynamics using directional Doppler technique. Part 1: Arteriovenous malformations. J. Neurosurg. 1979; 50: 145-151.

31. Nornes H., Grip A., Wikeby P.: Intraoperative evaluation of cerebral hemodynamics using directional Doppler technique. Part 2: Saccular aneurysms. J. Neurosurg. 1979; 50: 570-577.
32. Nornes H., Grip A.: Hemodynamic aspects of cerebral arteriovenous malformations. J. Neurosurg. 1980; 53: 456-464.
33. Hartley C.J., Hanley H.G., Lewis R.M., Cole J.S.: Synchronized pulsed Doppler blood flow and ultrasonic dimension measurements in conscious dogs. Ultrasound Med Biol. 1978; 4: 99-116.
34. Holen J., Aaslid R., Landmark K., Simonsen S.: Determination of pressure gradient in mitral stenosis with a non-invasive ultrasound Doppler technique. Acta Med. Scand. 1976; 199: 455-460.
35. Holen J., Aaslid R., Landmark K., Simonsen S., Østrem T.: Determination of effective orifice area in mitral stenosis from non-invasive ultrasound Doppler data and mitral flow rate. Acta Med. Scand. 1977; 201: 83-88.
36. Brubakk A.O., Angelsen B.A.J., Hatle L.: Diagnosis of valvular heart disease using transcutaneous Doppler ultrasound. Cardiovasc. Res. 1977; 11: 461-469.
37. Hatle L., Brubakk A., Tromsdal A., Angelsen B.: Non-invasive assessment of pressure drop in mitral stenosis by Doppler ultrasound. Br. Heart J. 1978; 40: 131-140.
38. Hatle L., Angelsen B.A., Tromsdal A.: Non-invasive assessment of aortic stenosis by Doppler ultrasound. Br. Heart J. 1980; 43: 284-292.
39. Skjærpe T., Hatle L.: Diagnosis and assessment of tricuspid regurgitation with Doppler ultrasound. Proceedings of Fourth Symposium on Echocardiology, Rotterdam, Martinus Nijhoff (Haag 1981).
40. Hatle L., Rokseth R.: Noninvasive diagnosis and assessment of ventriecular septal defect by Doppler ultrasound. Acta Med. Scand. 1981; Suppl. 645: 47-56.
41. Hatle L., Angelsen B.A.J., Tromsdal A.: Noninvasive estimation of pulmonary artery systolic pressure with Doppler ultrasound. Br. Heart J. 1981; 45: 157-165.
42. Reneman R.S., Clarke H.F., Simmons N., Spencer M.P.: In vivo comparison of electromagnetic and Doppler flowmeters: With special attention to the processing of analog Doppler flow signal. Cardiovasc. Res. 1973; 7: 557-566.
43. Baker D.W., Rubenstein G.A., Lorch G.S.: Pulsed Doppler echocardiography: Principles and applications. Am. J. Med. 1977; 63: 69-80.
44. Angelsen B.A.J.: Spectral estimation of a narrow-band Gaussian process from the distribution of the distance between adjacent zeros. IEEE Trans. Biomed. Eng. 1980; BME-27: 108-110.
45. Burckhardt C.B.: Comparison between spectrum and time interval histogram of ultrasound Doppler signals. Ultrasound Med. Biol. 1981; 7: 79-82.

2

Physics of Blood Flow

2.1 INTRODUCTION

This chapter describes the relationship between blood flow velocity and volumetric flow rate, the concepts of turbulent and laminar flows, and the relationship between the pressure and flow pulse waveforms in the heart and the arteries. These topics provide a background for how pathologies in the cardiovascular system affect ultrasonic Doppler measurements. Because the chapter is somewhat technical, the reader may prefer to read only the introduction before continuing to other parts of the book.

The *cardiac output,* which is the volume of blood pumped by the heart in a minute, is of special interest for evaluating the capacity of the heart. In the approximation of neglecting the flow in the coronary arteries, this can be obtained from the *volumetric flow rate* of blood in the ascending aorta by integration for one minute. If we integrate the flow rate during systole, we obtain the *cardiac stroke volume.* In aortic regurgitation, integration of the flow rate during diastole gives the *regurgitant volume.* The volumetric flow in peripheral vessels can indicate the capacity of the peripheral arteries for feeding the tissue.

With ultrasonic Doppler techniques, blood *velocities* can be measured. This is different from the volumetric flow rate of blood. One could say that volumetric flow rate is obtained by multiplying the velocity with the artery cross section, but this is an approximation because the velocity of the blood varies across the artery lumen. The velocity as a function of position in the vessel cross section is called the *velocity profile* in the vessel.

If we have a flat velocity profile (i.e., the blood velocity is constant across the lumen), the volumetric flow rate would be exactly equal to the velocity multiplied by the area of the artery lumen. Since the velocity varies across the lumen, we can define an *average velocity* over the artery cross section, $\bar{v}$, so that the volumetric flow rate, q, can be obtained as

$$q(t) = A \cdot \bar{v}(t) \tag{2.1}$$

where A is the area of the cross section. The t in the parentheses indicates that the variables can be a function of time. We term $\bar{v}(t)$ the *space average velocity* to differentiate it from the *time average velocity* to be discussed in the next section. The space average velocity can be a function of time.

To obtain volumetric flow rate with ultrasonic Doppler techniques, we must obtain both the mean velocity and the vessel cross section. If the angle between the ultrasonic beam and velocity direction is known and we have uniform insonification of the vessel, the mean velocity can be obtained from a mean frequency estimator (see Section 3.5B). However, these conditions are not easy to establish in the aorta; therefore, absolute values of flow rate are difficult to obtain. *Relative changes* in flow rate are more accessible with this method. This especially applies to changes in cardiac output as described in Chapter 7.

The reason why the blood velocity varies across the artery lumen is *viscous friction* between the blood and the vessel wall. The blood velocity is therefore zero at the wall and largest in the middle of the vessel. *Acceleration* of the blood when the heart is pumping also affects the velocity distribution in the artery by flattening the profile. The distribution depends therefore on both the viscosity and the acceleration of the blood.

When the blood velocity becomes sufficiently high, *turbulence* occurs, which causes the flow pattern to change from a regular varying appearance to a random, rapidly varying pattern. With flow disturbances in the heart, turbulent-like high velocity jets are often produced. The pulsed instruments that have been used have the limitation of frequency aliasing, by means of which positive and negative velocities are intermixed (see Sections 3.3B and 3.6). This has caused some confusion about the concept of turbulent flow, and too strong emphasis may have been put on using the degree of turbulence to characterize a lesion. We discuss turbulence in Section 2.3B.

The degree of some flow disturbances may be better characterized by the maximum velocity that occurs. A flow obstruction causes an increase in velocity, which requires a pressure drop along the flow path. For a *valve stenosis,* we can calculate the pressure drop across the valve as

$$\mathbf{p}_1 - \mathbf{p}_2 \approx \mathbf{4v}_2{}^2 \tag{2.2}$$

where v_2 is the maximum velocity in the stenotic jet. If v_2 is inserted in m/s, the pressure drop in mm Hg is obtained. By recording the maximum velocity in the jet with ultrasonic Doppler, one can obtain a *noninvasive* estimation of the pressure drop across a stenotic valve. A pressure drop is also required to overcome viscous friction and to produce acceleration of the flow. This is discussed in more detail in Section 2.4.

Since the heart is pumping periodically, both the pressure and the flow in the arteries have a pulsatile form. The elasticity of the vessel walls combines with the inertial forces in the blood so that the flow and pressure pulses travel with a certain *wave velocity* (5 to 10 m/s) similar to waves on a water surface. This causes transmission delays of the pulses along the arteries, and branching of the arteries causes reflections that change the form of the pulses. For this reason, the flow pulse in the aorta looks different than the flow pulse in a peripheral artery as discussed in Section 2.4.

2.2 VELOCITY AND VOLUMETRIC FLOW RATE

A. Velocity and Acceleration

Most people, at least those who have a driver's license, have an intuitive concept of velocity. The *instantaneous velocity* of a car can be read from the speedometer in km/h or mph. The *time* average velocity, $\tilde{v}$, between two places, A and B, can be found by dividing the distance, ℓ, between the two places by the time, t, used to drive between the two:

$$\tilde{v} = \frac{\ell}{t} \qquad (2.3)$$

It is evident that during the journey the instantaneous velocity, $v(t)$, is a function of time, and varies around the average velocity as one drives along.

The *time average* velocity defined here is not the same average as the *space average* of the velocity distribution across the vessel lumen defined in the previous section. This space average velocity in an artery is a function of time caused by the pumping of the heart. By averaging this over time, we obtain the time average of the space average velocity (see Section 3.5B).

The dimension of velocity is length/time. For the blood velocity it is practical to measure length in meters (m) or centimeters (cm) and time in seconds. Practical units for velocity, therefore, become m/s or cm/s. The SI unit* for length is m and for time it is seconds. The SI unit for velocity, therefore, becomes m/s.

To obtain the instantaneous velocity, we can measure the distance ($\triangle \ell$) the car moves in so short a time ($\triangle t$) that the velocity is approximately constant in this time interval. The velocity then can be calculated as

$$v \approx \frac{\triangle \ell}{\triangle t} \qquad (2.4)$$

If $\triangle t$ is made arbitrarily small, we obtain

$$v(t) = \frac{d\ell(t)}{dt} = \lim_{\triangle t \to 0} \frac{\triangle \ell}{\triangle t} \qquad (2.5)$$

where $\ell(t)$ is the distance the car traverses as a function of time. The velocity is thus the time derivative of this distance. This is illustrated in Figure 2.1a and b.

*SI = Système International

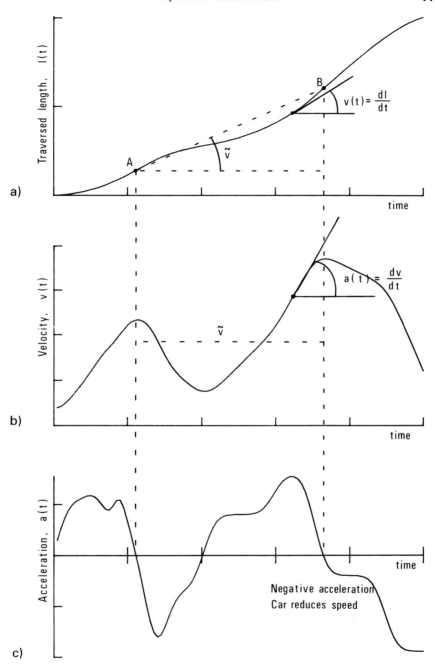

a)

b)

c)

Fig. 2–1. Relationship between traversed length, velocity, and acceleration.

The *acceleration* of the car is the rate of change of the velocity. Thus, the time derivative of the velocity is shown in Figure 2.1c:

$$\mathbf{a} = \frac{d\mathbf{v}}{dt} \qquad (2.6)$$

The dimension of acceleration is velocity/time or length/(time)^2. The SI unit for acceleration is, therefore, m/s^2.

We have seen that the velocity can be calculated from the traversed distance as a function of time through differentiation (see Equation 2.5). The traversed distance can be calculated from the velocity by integration:

$$\ell(t) = \int_0^t d\tau \, \mathbf{v}(\tau) \qquad (2.7)$$

The integral gives the area under the velocity curve from time zero to t. This is illustrated in Figure 2.2 for a constant velocity where the shaded area is equal to the traversed distance up to time (t). If the blood or car (or whatever object) moves with 1 m/s for 1 s, the traversed distance is

$$\ell = (1 \text{ m/s}) (1 \text{ s}) = 1 \text{ m} \qquad (2.8)$$

When we multiply velocity with time we obtain length.

Figure 2.3 shows how the traversed distance is obtained as the area under the velocity in the case of time-varying velocity. Note that the negative velocity reduces the traversed distance, i.e., the direction of movement is reversed.

If the *maximum velocity* in a blood vessel is integrated, we obtain the distance traversed by the small blood volume which has this maximum velocity. If the *space average velocity* is integrated, we obtain a fictitious distance that the blood would have traversed if all blood moved with this average velocity. If the space average velocity in the ascending aorta is integrated for one cardiac cycle and multiplied with the cross-sectional area of the ascending aorta, cardiac *stroke volume* is obtained, according to the discussion in Section 2.1.

Both velocity and acceleration have direction and magnitude. Such a variable is called *vector valued*. This is indicated by an arrow over the letter $\vec{v}$. It has special significance for ultrasonic Doppler measurements of velocity since it is the *component* of the velocity vector along the ultrasonic beam that produces the Doppler shift. This is illustrated in Figure 2.4.

Combining Equations 2.3 and 2.7 shows how the time average of the velocity over the interval (0, t) can be calculated from the instantaneous velocity:

$$\tilde{\mathbf{v}} = \frac{\ell(t)}{t} = \frac{1}{t} \int_0^t d\tau \, \mathbf{v}(\tau) \qquad (2.9)$$

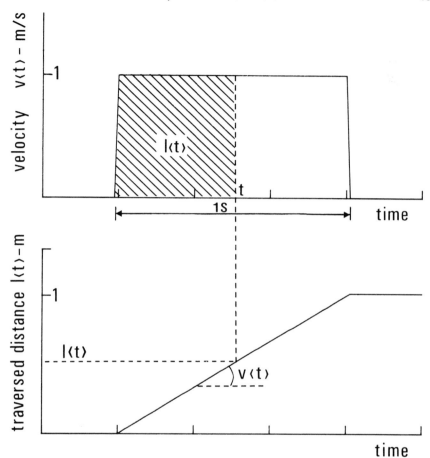

Fig. 2–2. Calculation of traversed distance from the velocity in the case of constant velocity.

B. Volumetric Flow Rate

As already noted in the introduction, the volumetric flow rate of the blood is a different concept than velocity. This is important to notice since ultrasonic Doppler techniques measure blood velocity and not volumetric flow rate.

The time average volumetric flow rate in an artery ($\bar{q}$) can be measured if we cut across the artery and measure the volume (V) of blood that flows into a cup in the time (t). We then obtain

$$\bar{q}(t) = \frac{V}{t} \qquad\qquad (2.10)$$

When the instantaneous flow rate varies with time, it can be measured

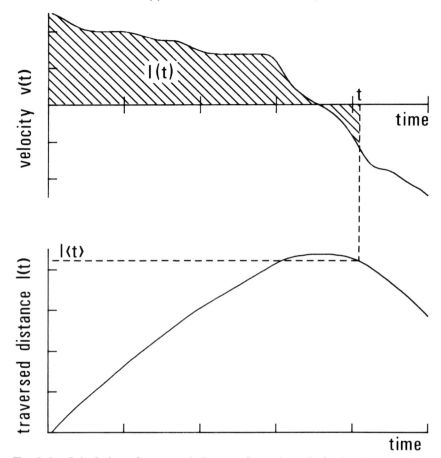

Fig. 2–3. Calculation of traversed distance from the velocity in the case of time varying velocity. Note that the negative velocity reduces the traversed distance, i.e., the direction of movement is reversed.

approximately from the volume ($\triangle$V) that flows into the cup in a small time interval ($\triangle$t). This time interval should be so short that the flow rate is approximately constant during the interval. We then obtain

$$q(t) \approx \frac{\triangle V(t)}{\triangle t} \qquad\qquad (2.11)$$

In the limit that $\triangle t \to 0$ we obtain, in a similar way as for the velocity,

$$q(t) = \frac{dV(t)}{dt} = \lim_{\triangle t \to 0} \frac{\triangle V}{\triangle t} \qquad\qquad (2.12)$$

The volumetric flow rate is thus the *rate of change* of the *volume* of blood in the cup as a function of time. For the flow rate we are concerned with the *volume* which flows into the cup, whereas for velocity we are concerned with the *distance* which is traversed in the time (Δt). When the velocity is integrated, we obtain traversed distance. Similarly, when flow rate is integrated, we obtain the volume of blood in the cup. The same volume has passed through the artery cross section during this time. The integral

$$V(t) = \int_0^t d\tau\, q(\tau) \tag{2.13}$$

is then the volume which has passed the artery cross section in the time interval (0, t).

The dimension of flow rate is volume/time. In SI units volume is measured in cubic meters (m^3) so that the SI unit for volumetric flow rate is m^3/s. A more practical unit for blood flow measurements is cubic centimeters/second (cm^3/s) or $m\ell/s$.

If we have a flow rate of 100 $m\ell/s$, the volume of blood that passes an artery cross section per second is

$$100\,(m\ell/s) \cdot 1s = 100\ m\ell \tag{2.14}$$

Now assume that all blood in the vessel has a constant velocity (v), i.e., we have a *flat* time-constant velocity profile. The volume of blood that flows through a cross section of the artery in the time, t, takes the shape of a

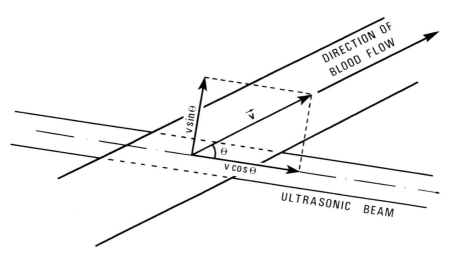

Fig. 2–4. **Decomposition of a velocity vector into a component parallel to the beam and at an angle of 90° to the beam.**

cylinder with length, vt, and cross sectional area, A. This is illustrated in Figure 2.5a. The volume is then

$$V(t) = A \cdot v \cdot t \tag{2.15}$$

and the flow rate becomes

$$q = \frac{V(t)}{t} = A \cdot v \tag{2.16}$$

i.e., area times velocity.

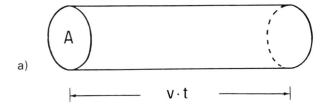

a)

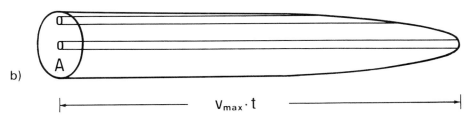

b)

Fig. 2–5. Volume of blood passing through a vessel cross section in time (t) for a flat velocity profile (a) and a parabolic profile (b) with the same volumetric flow rate.

When the velocity varies across the vessel lumen, i.e., the velocity profile is not flat, the arterial lumen can be divided into small areas, $\triangle A$, so that the velocity is approximately constant over each area. The blood flowing through different areas then produces cylinders of different volumes ($\triangle A \cdot v \cdot t$) since v varies between different areas. This is illustrated in Figure 2.5b. The total blood volume that has passed the cross section in a time, t, is then the sum of the small volumes passing through each of the small areas. In this way the volumetric flow rate can be calculated from the velocity profile as shown in more detail in Appendix A.

The *space average* or *mean velocity* in a vessel is defined as the velocity of a flat profile that produces the same volumetric flow rate:

$$q(t) = A \cdot \tilde{v}(t) \tag{2.17}$$

An obstruction in the flow path, such as a stenotic valve, produces a reduction in the area (A) which is followed by an increase in the velocity to maintain the volumetric flow rate (q). This acceleration is called *convective* since it is caused by the convection or streaming of the blood from one part of the vessel with a low velocity to another part with a higher velocity.

2.3   VISCOSITY, VELOCITY PROFILE, AND TURBULENT FLOW

A.   Viscosity and Laminar Velocity Profiles

When two neighboring elements of a fluid flow with different velocities, there are frictional forces between the two caused by the viscosity of the fluid. For a fluid with high viscosity (syrup), the frictional forces are higher than for a fluid with low viscosity (water).

The blood is a mixture of solid elements (the cells) and the plasma, which is a liquid. The viscous friction in the blood is, therefore, fairly complex. However, for the velocity gradients that exist in arteries with a radius above 1 mm, blood behaves approximately as a pure liquid. There is then a linear relationship between the viscous sheer tension and the velocity gradient. A fluid that has a linear viscosity is called a *Newtonian fluid* and the viscosity can be described by a coefficient of viscosity, μ. The dimension of the coefficient of viscosity is Ns/m^2 = Pas (Pascal seconds). N (Newton) = kg m/s^2 is the SI unit for force and Pa (Pascal) = N/m^2 is the SI unit for tension. The viscosity of normal blood[1] is approximately

$$\mu \approx 10^{-2} \text{ Pas} \tag{2.18}$$

This value can vary, especially with certain diseases.

The viscosity of the fluid tends to smooth the fluid motion. At low velocities the fluid elements flow along regular lines. The flow is then termed *laminar*. In a straight circular tube at a far distance from the inlet of the tube, time-steady flow of a Newtonian fluid produces a parabolic velocity profile, as shown in Figure 2.6. Nonlinear viscous fluids give other profiles. In the cardiac chambers the velocity profiles have a fairly complex shape, e.g., flow direction changes dramatically from left ventricular inlet to outlet. Although whirls and eddies are found in the chambers, the flow is still laminar in most normal and many pathologic situations. A review of different profiles is given by McDonald.[2]

The viscous friction produces a flow resistance. A pressure drop along the vessel is required to drive a steady flow. This is described by *Poiseuille's law*:

$$q = R^{-1} \triangle p \tag{2.19}$$

For a parabolic profile the viscous resistance, R, is

$$R = \frac{8\mu\ell}{\pi a^4} \tag{2.20}$$

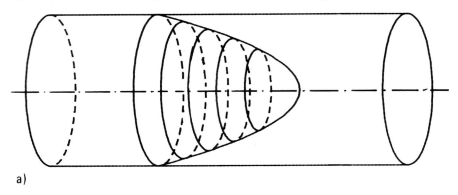

a)

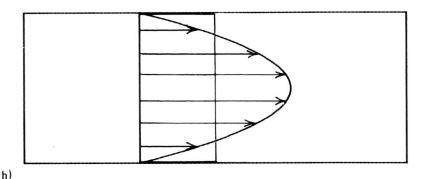

b)

Fig. 2–6. Parabolic velocity profile in a vessel in three dimensions (a) and schematically in two dimensions (b). The latter also shows the flat profile that gives the same volumetric flow. This gives the space average or mean velocity.

where ℓ is the length of the vessel where we have the pressure drop ($\triangle p$). The radius of the vessel lumen is a. The resistance thus becomes larger as the vessel diminishes in size. For blunt profiles a larger value of R is found. Equation 2.19 is equivalent to Ohm's law for electrical current.

Acceleration of the blood flow adds a *flat* component to the velocity profile. For this reason the velocity profile in the aorta, where the flow is strongly pulsatile due to heart pumping, is fairly flat. This is illustrated in Figure 2.7a. Note that the diastolic flow is approximately zero owing to the large compliance of the aorta. Less acceleration is required to produce a flat profile in a large artery such as the aorta than in a smaller peripheral artery because the viscous resistance is larger in the smaller artery.

In a peripheral artery there can be substantial diastolic flow if the peripheral resistance is small compared to the artery compliance. This can be found

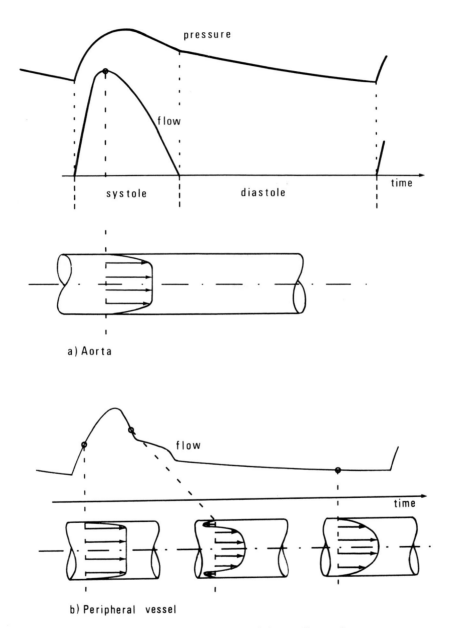

Fig. 2–7. **Velocity profiles at various phases of the cardiac cycle.**

in the internal carotid artery, the renal artery, and in cases of vasodilatation (e.g., when arteries feed the muscles during muscular work). The flow is then less strongly accelerated, and the profile is nearly parabolic, as illustrated in Figure 2.7b. In the acceleration phase in the systole, the profile is flatter. In the retardation phase in late systole there can even be negative velocities close to the artery walls because the retardation adds a flat negative component to the profile. Since the velocity is small near the walls before the deacceleration, velocities in the opposite direction are found.

In a vein the flow has very small accelerations; therefore, a parabolic profile is found.

When a vessel branches off from a larger one, the profile near the inlet is flat, regardless of whether the flow is accelerated or not. If the flow is steady, the flat profile develops into a parabolic profile after a distance of 5 to 10 vessel diameters from the inlet. This is illustrated in Figure 2.8. If the flow is accelerated, a flat profile is found all along the tube.

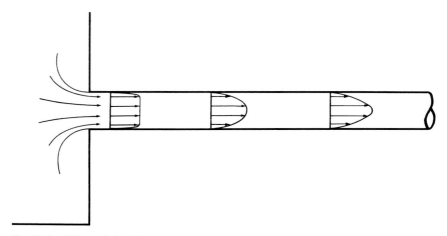

Fig. 2–8.   Effect of the inlet geometry on the velocity profile.

In summary, we have the following:

1. The velocity profile is determined by geometric factors (such as shape of vessel and distance from the inlet), viscosity, and acceleration.

2. In a circular vessel far from the inlet, time steady flow produces a parabolic profile. At the inlet the profile is flat.

3. If the flow is accelerated, the profile is flattened. Less acceleration is required to flatten the profile in a large vessel, such as the aorta, than in a smaller peripheral vessel where viscous resistance is higher.

B. Turbulent Flow

As the velocity increases, the laminar regularity of the flow changes. The flow changes from laminar to *turbulent*.[3] In a turbulent flow, the velocity of the fluid elements passing through a particular point in the vessel changes rapidly with time, although the volumetric flow rate across the whole vessel lumen must have a smooth variation with time.

In turbulence each fluid element also has velocity components transverse to the tube axis. The velocity as a whole can be decomposed into a sum of two terms: one slowly varying term and one *random* rapidly varying term. The slowly varying term has no components transverse to the vessel axis, and the random term produces no net flow across the vessel lumen. This slowly varying term then represents a turbulent velocity profile which, for instance, can be obtained by using a hot film anemometer and low pass filtering of the output. The turbulent velocity profile is flatter than the laminar velocity profile.

Owing to the transverse velocity components, the interchange of energy between the different points in the cross section is much larger for turbulent than for laminar flow. In laminar flow the only interchange of energy is caused by viscous friction. The random velocity component causes an additional energy loss in turbulent flow. This is observed as an additional resistance to flow, arising from *Reynolds stresses*. The flow resistance, therefore, increases as the flow changes from laminar to turbulent.

The transition between laminar and turbulent flow occurs over a diffuse range of flow rates rather than at a sharp value of the flow rate. At low flow rates, the laminar flow is stable so that any disturbance away from laminar flow decays with time. As the flow rate increases, the laminar velocity profile becomes unstable and a small disturbance (e.g., by external vibration) away from the laminar profile develops into full turbulent flow. If the external disturbance is minimized and the vessel wall is smooth, laminar flow can be obtained at flow rates that otherwise would produce turbulent flow.

The Reynolds number, R_E, is often used to characterize the flow:

$$R_E = \frac{\rho dv}{\mu} \qquad\qquad (2.21)$$

where

ρ = mass density in kg/m^3

d = vessel diameter in m

v = velocity in m/s

μ = viscosity in Pa · s = kg/sm

R_E is a dimensionless number. For $R_E > 2000$, turbulent flow tends to develop. However, in carefully prepared experiments, laminar flow has been obtained for R_E much higher than this ($\sim$50,000).

Typical values for blood are

$\mu = 10^{-2}$ **Pa · s**	$\rho = 1.06 \cdot 10^3$ **kg/m³**	$v = 1$ **m/s**
aorta:	$d = 2.5$ **cm**	$R_E = 2650$
peripheral vessel:	$d = .5$ **cm**	$R_E = 530$

We can express the Reynolds number by the volumetric flow rate $q = v/A$.

$$R_E = \frac{\rho dq}{\mu A} \tag{2.22}$$

If an obstruction is in the artery, the volumetric flow is constant (see Section 2.2), but the area (A) decreases. This increases R_E so that turbulence can be caused.

In the heart one can have high velocity blood jets in stenotic valves, valve regurgitations, and septal defects. The high velocity jet streams into a wide region of blood flowing with lower velocity.

It is unclear whether the jet is turbulent or not. In vitro flow studies indicate that the flow is often laminar in the obstruction. In the friction between the jet and the slowly flowing blood, turbulent-like eddies are formed, and later on the jet core itself develops into a turbulent-like flow. This has been partially confirmed by in vivo measurements using 1 MHz pulsed ultrasound and doubling of the range velocity product as discussed in Section 3.6. A narrow-band Doppler spectrum has then been found occasionally in the obstruction.

2.4 BLOOD DYNAMICS

A. Pressure Velocity Relationships

The driving force for the blood flow through the vessel is the pressure drop along the vessel. For *time steady* flow in a tube with constant cross section, the *viscous friction* outbalances the pressure drop

$$\triangle p = Rq \tag{2.23}$$

where R is the viscous resistance in the vessel. For parabolic flow, R is given in Equation 2.20, while other values are obtained for other profiles. This is analogous to Ohm's law for electric current and voltage.

If the blood flow is *accelerated,* additional pressure drop is required to overcome the *inertial forces.* In addition to this, a change of the flow cross section causes convective acceleration as discussed in connection with Equation 2.2. The pressure drop which is required for the convective acceleration is

$$p_1 - p_2 = \frac{1}{2}\rho\,(v_2^2 - v_1^2) \tag{2.24}$$

The subscripts 1 and 2 indicate two positions along the flow lines. This is shown in Figure 2.9. ρ is the mass density of the blood. Equation 2.24 gives the pressure drop as the increase in kinetic energy per unit volume of the fluid. This is similar to the increase in kinetic energy of a falling stone in the gravitational field. The pressure drop is related solely to the increase in velocity and is independent of the size of the orifice (assuming viscous friction can be neglected). This is analogous to a large and small stone having the same increase in velocity in a gravitational field.

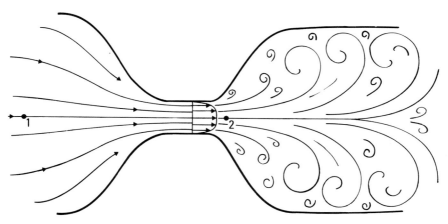

Fig. 2–9. Schematic flow through an obstruction.

The equation is useful for calculating the pressure drop across a stenotic valve or a septal defect. The velocity in front of the jet (v_1) is usually much smaller than the maximum velocity in the jet (v_2). Therefore, we can neglect v_1^2 compared to v_2^2. Inserting $\rho = 1.06 \cdot 10^3$ kg/m³ we obtain approximately

$$p_1 - p_2 = 4v_2^2 \tag{2.25}$$

where v_2 in m/s gives the pressure drop in mm Hg.

The maximum velocity in the jet can be measured noninvasively using ultrasonic Doppler techniques. By means of Equation 2.25, the pressure drop across a valve stenosis or a septal defect can be obtained noninvasively.

This was first accomplished by Holen, et al.[4,5] and was later applied by Hatle, et al.[6,7]

Equation 2.24 only gives the part of the pressure drop which comes from convective acceleration. We have neglected viscous friction and the inertial pressure drop which comes from a change of the flow rate itself with time. These terms can be included, and we obtain the *Bernoulli equation:*

$$\mathbf{p}_1 - \mathbf{p}_2 = \underbrace{\frac{1}{2}\rho\,(\mathbf{v}_2{}^2 - \mathbf{v}_1{}^2)}_{\substack{\text{convective}\\\text{acceleration}}} + \underbrace{\rho\int_1^2 \frac{d\vec{\mathbf{v}}}{dt}\,d\vec{\mathbf{s}}}_{\substack{\text{flow}\\\text{acceleration}}} + \underbrace{\mathbf{R}\,(\vec{\mathbf{v}})}_{\substack{\text{viscous}\\\text{friction}}} \qquad (2.26)$$

The viscous friction depends not only on the local velocity, but on the whole velocity profile, since it is caused by friction between neighboring fluid elements. The velocity profile in a stenotic valve is flat, as shown in Figure 2.9. This indicates that viscous friction in the center of the lumen can be neglected, which was confirmed by in vitro experiments of Holen, et al. who showed that the pressure drop could be calculated from Equation 2.25 accurately for orifices of 8 mm diameter.[4] When the orifice diameter was reduced to 3.5 mm, the pressure drop was underestimated using Equation 2.25. The underestimation was larger for the smaller velocities (< 3 m/s), and the accuracy was acceptable for velocities above this limit. For a 1.5 mm orifice, the estimated pressure drop was about half the actual pressure drop. Since actual orifice diameters are above 3.5 mm, this together with other findings[5-8] indicates that Equation 2.25 is valuable for clinical applications.

The second term only contributes during valve opening and closure where the flow acceleration is high. It causes a delay between the pressure drop curve and the velocity curve. The pressure drop calculated from the velocity by Equation 2.25 is, therefore, somewhat delayed from the true curve as indicated in Figure 2.10 for typical waveforms found in mitral stenosis.

For a stenotic mitral valve, the velocity increases from 0 to 2 m/s in .1 s during the valve opening. This gives an approximate acceleration of

$$\frac{dv}{dt} = \frac{2}{.1} = 20 \text{ m/s}^2 \qquad (2.27)$$

Assume that we measure the pressure drop over a distance of $\ell = 3$ cm. An estimate of the magnitude of the second term is

$$\rho\frac{dv}{dt}\,\ell = 636\,\frac{N}{m^2} \sim 5 \text{ mm Hg} \qquad (2.28)$$

Because 2 m/s produces a convective pressure drop of 16 mm Hg, for clinical purposes this delay is negligible.[4]

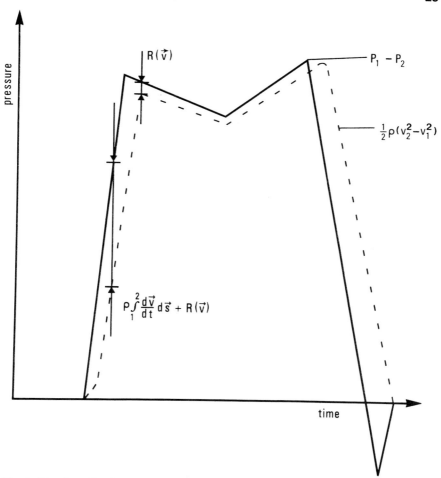

Fig. 2–10. **Contribution of the different terms in Equation 2.23 to the pressure drop in mitral stenosis.**

For aortic stenosis we have found a larger delay between the jet velocity and the pressure drop.[6] Assume that the velocity changes from 0 to 5 m/s during .1 s at the opening of the valve in aortic stenosis. This gives an approximate acceleration of

$$\frac{dv}{dt} = \frac{5}{.1} = 50 \text{ m/s}^2 \qquad (2.29)$$

Assume that we measure the pressure drop over 5 cm here, since the aortic jet is longer than the mitral jet. We can then give an estimate of the magnitude of the second term in Equation 2.26.

$$\rho \frac{dv}{dt}\, \ell = 2650\ \frac{N}{m^2} \sim 20\ mm\ Hg \tag{2.30}$$

This produces a sizable lag between velocity and pressure drop and is probably the main reason for the lag in the noninvasive estimation of pressure drop in aortic stenosis discussed in Chapter 5. Murgo, et al. have performed precise measurements of pulsatile flow and pressure drop across normal aortic valves.[9] The lags they have found indicate that Equation 2.30 gives a reasonable value for aortic stenosis.

Despite the inaccuracy during early systole, Equation 2.25 gives a clinically acceptable estimate of the pressure drop in aortic stenosis.

B. Transmission of Pressure and Flow Pulses

An in-depth treatment of the transmission of pressure and flow pulses is given by McDonald.[2] The following is a review of some basic points relevant to ultrasonic blood velocity measurements.

The vessel walls are elastic so that the area of the vessel lumen increases with increasing pressure. When the heart ejects its stroke volume into the aorta, the total volume of the aorta increases due to the increase in pressure, so that most of the ejected blood remains in the aorta during systole and flows to the periphery during diastole. The aorta is thus a reservoir which smooths the action of the heart's pulsatile pumping.

We can model the aorta with an elastic balloon called the Windkessel model (Figure 2.11). The flow into the aorta when the heart contracts is composed of two terms. The first, which is called the compliant term, produces a volume expansion of the aorta itself. The other represents the outflow from the aorta to the periphery and is called the conductive term.

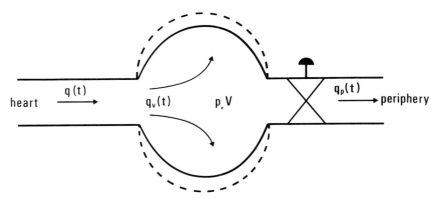

Fig. 2–11.   Windkessel model of the aorta. The dotted line indicates the balloon during systole, and the solid line indicates the balloon at end-diastole.

The pressure-volume relationship of the aortic balloon is

$$V = Cp \qquad (2.31)$$

where V is the volume of the aorta, p is the aortic pressure, and C is a constant of proportionality called the volume compliance of the aorta. Since the compliant flow rate, q_v, represents the volume expansion of the aorta, we obtain the following from Equation 2.12:

$$q_v(t) = \frac{dV}{dt} = C\frac{dp}{dt} \qquad (2.32)$$

It is, then, proportional to the derivative of the pressure waveform. The conductive outflow, q_p, of the aorta is proportional to the aortic pressure

$$q_p(t) = G_p p \qquad (2.33)$$

where G_p is a constant of proportionality called the peripheral conductance. $G_p = R_p^{-1}$ where R_p is the peripheral resistance. The total inflow to the aorta is then

$$q(t) = q_v(t) + q_p(t) = C\frac{dp}{dt} + G_p p \qquad (2.34)$$

The flow of blood in arteries has a close analogy to transmission of electrical signals. The inflow of blood into the aorta can thus be represented by an electrical analogue circuit as shown in Figure 2.12. The capacitor, C, represents the volume compliance of the aorta and the resistor, R_p, represents the peripheral outflow. The capacitor is charged during systole by the ejection from the heart and is discharged through R_p during diastole. This causes an approximately exponential decay of the aortic pressure during diastole.

The inertial forces of the moving blood combine with the compliance of the vessel so that the pressure pulse travels toward the periphery as a wave similar to waves on a water surface. A better analogy, for those who understand the concept, is electrical waves on an electrical transmission line. The wave velocity is 5 to 10 m/s. The branching of the aorta causes reflections which are found as a notch in the velocity curve as illustrated in Figure 2.13. The negative flow is required to close the valve.

During systole, the first term is much larger than the last term so that we approximately obtain

$$q(t) \approx C\frac{dp}{dt} \qquad (2.35)$$

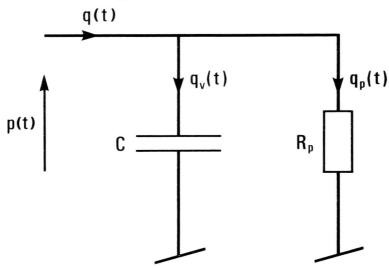

Fig. 2–12.   **Electrical analogue of the Windkessel model.**

The conductive term is usually so small in the ascending aorta that the flow can be neglected in diastole, as indicated in Figure 2.13.

As we move along the aorta, the diastolic flow can increase. For example, if one is performing muscular work with the arms, there is a diastolic flow toward the arms in the abdominal aorta and even as far distal as the femoral artery. The aorta (and parts of the legs) then functions as a reservoir that is

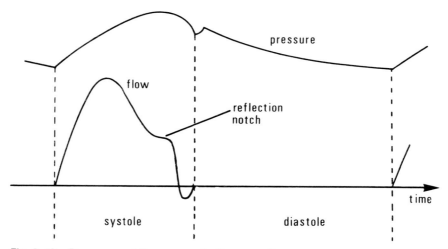

Fig. 2–13.   **Pressure and flow curves in the ascending aorta.**

filled during systole and supplies the arms with blood during diastole. Similarly, if one is performing muscular work with the legs, there is a diastolic flow toward the legs in the descending aorta.

The wave transmission causes a propagation delay of the pressure and flow pulses as they travel towards the periphery. A typical delay is 100 m/s from the ascending aorta to the femoral artery as shown in Figure 2.14. Because of the tapering of the aorta and reflections from the periphery, the pulses also change shape, and even the maximum systolic pressure increases, as indicated in Figure 2.14.

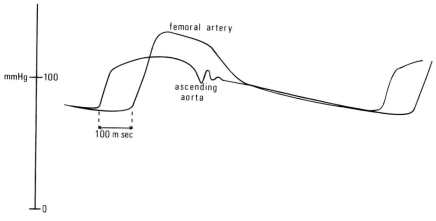

Fig. 2–14.   Pressure waveforms in the ascending aorta and the femoral artery.

The flow pulse becomes steeper and reflections can cause negative and positive flow oscillations in the diastole as indicated in Figure 2.15. This shows typical waveforms found in the femoral, the brachial, and similar arteries during rest. If muscular work increases, the last term in Equation 2.34 can become important during diastole. We then obtain a flow waveform similar to the one shown in Figure 2.16. Since the conductive term in Equation 2.34 is proportional to the pressure, we see that the flow waveform has become more similar to the pressure waveform.

The type of flow waveform in Figure 2.16 is found when the conductant flow is larger than the compliant flow, seen from the location of measurement. This occurs in the internal carotid artery, the renal artery, and other arteries when at vasodilatation.

If there is a stenosis in the artery, this dampens the pulsatility of both the pressure and the flow wave. The resistance in the stenosis, combined with the distal compliance in the artery, functions as a low pass filter. The venous flow velocities do not have the same type of pulsatile shape as in arteries. They have a much slower variation with time since the driving force is

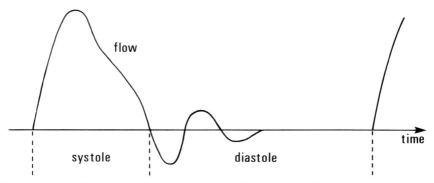

Fig. 2–15. Oscillatory flow waveform in a peripheral artery during rest.

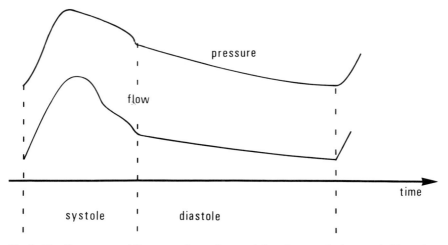

Fig. 2–16. Pressure and flow waveforms in a peripheral artery during work. Note that conductive flow is significant in diastole.

mainly caused by muscular pumping and breathing. Because of the low acceleration, the velocity profile is parabolic.

In summary, we have the following:

1. The action of the arterial tree on the form of the pressure and flow waveforms in arteries is determined by three factors: peripheral conductance, vessel compliance, and blood inertia. The last two factors combine to produce a wave nature of the pulse transmission which causes reflections.

This changes the waveforms and can even cause an oscillatory behavior of the flow pulse as one moves from the heart toward the periphery.

2. The compliant part of the flow is proportional to the time derivative of the pressure wave. This is the main part of the flow in the ascending aorta.

3. The conductive part is proportional to the pressure itself. It causes the flow waveform to become more similar to the pressure waveform in the arteries that go to the organs and the brain, and also in the arteries that feed muscles during work.

The contractility of the heart affects the waveforms in the arteries, mostly close to the ventricles (left and right) since the influence of transmission line effects on the pulse waveforms increases as one moves towards the periphery. A high contractility gives a fast rise to the waveforms in early systole. The contraction of the heart is also influenced by the pressure it pumps against. The flow waveforms in the pulmonary artery and the aorta are, therefore, different since the pulmonary pressure is normally lower than the aortic pressure, as demonstrated in Figures 4.9 and 4.10. In pulmonary hypertension the pulmonary waveform becomes more similar to the aortic waveform, as shown in Figure 5.72. For the flow through the valves and in the cavities of the heart, the flow waveforms are actively controlled by the muscle contraction and valve opening and closure. Examples of these waveforms are given in Chapters 4 and 5.

REFERENCES

1. Fung Y.C.: Biomechanics: A survey of the blood flow problem. Adv. Appl. Mech. 1971; 11: 65-130.
2. McDonald D.A.: Blood flow in arteries. London, Edward Arnold, 1974.
3. Caro C.G., Pedley T.J., Schroter R.C., Seed W.A.: The mechanics of the circulation. Oxford, Oxford University Press 1978.
4. Holen J., Aaslid R., Landmark K., Simonsen S., Østrem T.: Determination of effective orifice area in mitral stenosis from non-invasive ultrasound Doppler data and mitral flow rate. Acta Med. Scand. 1977; 201: 83-88.
5. Holen J., Aaslid R., Landmark K., Simonsen S.: Determination of pressure gradient in mitral stenosis with a non-invasive ultrasound Doppler technique. Acta Med. Scand. 1976; 199: 455-460.
6. Hatle L., Brubakk A.O., Tromsdal A., Angelsen B.: Noninvasive assessment of pressure drop in mitral stenosis by Doppler ultrasound. Br. Heart J. 1978; 40: 131-140.
7. Hatle L., Angelsen B.A., Tromsdal A.: Non-invasive assessment of aortic stenosis by Doppler ultrasound. Br. Heart J. 1980; 43: 284-292.
8. Skjærpe T., Hatle L.: Diagnosis and assessment of tricuspid regurgitation with Doppler ultrasound. Proceedings of Fourth Symposium on Echocardiology, Rotterdam, Martinus Nijhoff (Haag 1981), 299-304.
9. Murgo J.P., Altobelli S.A., Dorethy J.F., Logsdon J.R., McGranahan G.M.: Normal ventricular ejection dynamics in man during rest and exercise. *In:* Physiologic Principles of Heart Sounds and Murmurs. Edited by Leon S.F., Shaver J.A. Dallas, American Heart Association 1975; 92-101.

3

Blood Velocity Measurements Using The
Doppler Effect of Backscattered Ultrasound

3.1 ULTRASONIC TRANSDUCERS AND ACOUSTIC FIELD

As already noted in the introduction, ultrasound, like audible sound, is acoustic waves, but with frequencies above the audible range. If the frequency, f, is increased, the wavelength, λ, is reduced by the inverse proportion

$$\lambda = \frac{c}{f} \tag{3.1}$$

where c is the velocity of sound ($\approx$1560 m/s in biological tissue).

When the wavelength is reduced, the sound tends to move along straight lines. Low-frequency sound, like the bass in an orchestra, bends around corners. However, the treble sound from a loudspeaker is more directive. How well the treble sound is heard depends on where in the room one is standing.

The phenomenon of sound bending around corners is called *diffraction*. It is caused by the wave nature of the sound and is found with all types of waves (e.g., with light), and occurs when the geometrical dimensions of the system become comparable to the wavelength. For ultrasound in biological tissue we have

$$f = \ \ 2 \text{ MHz} \qquad \lambda = .78 \text{ mm}$$
$$f = 10 \text{ MHz} \qquad \lambda = .156 \text{ mm}$$

A typical 2 MHz transducer has a cylindrical shape with a 15-mm diameter. The front face vibrates like a piston with approximately uniform amplitude across the face. The diameter of the transducer is then approximately 20 wavelengths. With this relative dimension of the transducer, diffraction effects are seen, but the sound for a first approximation moves in straight lines. A lens can be used to focus the sound in a similar way as for light.

However, the minimum diameter of the focus is limited by diffraction effects. This is illustrated in Figure 3.1, which shows a Schlieren photograph of the acoustic field in water from a transducer. With this technique the acoustic field is visualized using interaction between light and the acoustic wave. The focus is not sharp, and two beams of sound outside the central lobe are seen.

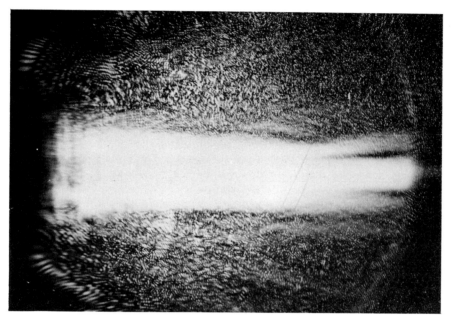

Fig. 3–1. Schlieren photograph of acoustic field from a transducer.

These are called side lobes. There are several of them at increasing angles from the axis, but with rapidly decreasing intensity. Therefore, only the first ones in the figure can be seen. Because of the axial symmetry, the side lobes actually form a skirt around the main lobe.

The diffraction effects make the edges of the beam less clear, so that the region where the blood velocity is observed has blurred boundaries. If we define the diameter, d_{f0}, of the focus by the zero of the intensity between the main lobe and the side lobe, we obtain

$$d_{f0} = 2.44\lambda \frac{\ell_f}{d} \tag{3.2}$$

where ℓ_f is the focal length and d is the diameter of the transducer. For d = 15 mm and ℓ_f = 8 cm at 2 MHz, we obtain d_f = 10 mm. Owing to the diffuse boundary of the main lobe, this is not an obvious definition of the diameter. If we define the diameter, d_{f1}, where the intensity of the transmitted beam is reduced to one-tenth of the maximum intensity in the central lobe, we obtain

$$\mathbf{d_{f1}} = \mathbf{1.72\lambda} \,\frac{\ell_f}{\mathbf{d}} \tag{3.3}$$

For the same transducer as just mentioned, we obtain d_{f1} = 7.15 mm. *We should note that erroneous signals from the side lobes can also be picked up.*

The sensitivity of the receiving transducer varies with the position of the scatterer. We thus obtain a *sensitivity pattern* of the receiving transducer which is the same as the field pattern when the transducer is transmitting. If the same transducer is used for transmission and reception, the amplitude of the backscattered signal as a function of the scatterer position is then proportional to the square (transmission and reception multiplied) of the amplitude of the transmitted acoustic wave at the location of the scatterer.

3.2   THE SCATTERING OF ULTRASOUND FROM BLOOD

It is mainly the red cells that scatter the ultrasound from the blood. The total signal is then the sum of the contributions from the different scatterers located at different positions. Two scatterers can be located so that the signal from the two cancel each other (destructive interference) or so that they add constructively (constructive interference). Because of destructive interference, a completely constant concentration of red cells produces little backscattered signal. When the cell concentration varies in space, the scattering is much stronger.

Therefore, it is more convenient to consider the scattering as occurring from the fluctuations in the cell concentration rather than from the individual cells as such.[1] The elementary scatterer is defined as a volume element of blood which is so small that the velocity profile within the element is practically constant. This volume element then produces a Doppler shift in frequency similar to a single particle scatterer. The scattering intensity is then proportional to

$$<\triangle n^2> \triangle V \tag{3.4}$$

where $\triangle V$ is the volume of the element and $<\triangle n^2>$ is the mean square fluctuation of the red cells in the blood. $<\triangle n^2> = <(n - n_0)^2>$ where n is the local cell concentration, n_0 is the mean cell concentration (time average), and $< >$ denotes averaging. The scatterers are thus distributed throughout the blood and the total backscattered signal power is, therefore, proportional to the total volume of scatterers observed. For a pulsed Doppler instrument, the signal/noise ratio increases with the size of the range cell. This leads to a different optimization of an ultrasonic Doppler instrument compared to an amplitude imaging instrument, which is discussed in Section 3.7 and Appendix B.

Turbulence increases the scattering since it increases $<\Delta n^2>$. The small eddies in the turbulence create a centrifugal effect which separates plasma and blood cells, owing to their difference in mass density. This increases the fluctuation which gives an increased scattering from the blood. This is probably the reason why jets in the blood cause stronger signals than ordinary flows.

3.3 BASIC PRINCIPLES OF ULTRASONIC DOPPLER TECHNIQUES

The principle of ultrasonic Doppler blood velocity measurement is schematically illustrated in Figure 3.2. We can use both *continuous wave* (CW) and *pulsed wave* (PW) ultrasound. The two techniques have special advantages and drawbacks. These are listed in Table 3.1.

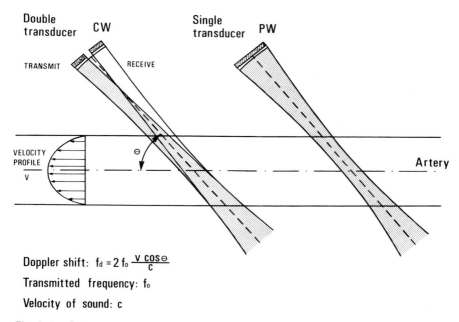

Doppler shift: $f_d = 2 f_0 \dfrac{V \cos\Theta}{c}$

Transmitted frequency: f_0

Velocity of sound: c

Fig. 3–2.   Principles of ultrasonic Doppler blood velocity measurement.

In the PW mode we obtain *range resolution,* i.e., we can measure the velocity in a small range cell at a variable depth along the ultrasonic beam. The size of the range cell depends on the instrument and the frequency. However, in the PW mode there is a *limit on the maximum velocity* that can be measured. This is a drawback of the technique.

Table 3.1 Comparison Between PW and CW Techniques

PW Technique	CW Technique
Range resolution (advantage).	No range resolution (disadvantage).
Limit on maximum velocity (disadvantage).	No limit on maximum measurable velocity (advantage).
Possible range ambiguity (to be aware of).	Poorer sensitivity than PW caused by diffraction from smaller transducers (disadvantage).

The CW mode has no range resolution, but at the same time there is no limit on the maximum velocity that can be measured. The two techniques, therefore, complement each other, and an instrument that combines the two is a much more powerful tool for diagnosis than a single PW or CW instrument.

If we increase the pulse repetition frequency in the PW mode so much that more than one pulse is traveling in the heart at each instant of time, there may be a problem with *range ambiguity*. This can, however, be used to measure higher velocities and is discussed subsequently.

A. Continuous Wave (CW) Doppler Technique

In the CW mode, continuous ultrasound is radiated towards the vessel from a transmitting transducer. The ultrasound is backscattered from the blood with a change in frequency given by the Doppler equation (Equation 3.5). The backscattered sound is picked up by a receiver transducer as illustrated to the left in Figure 3.2. The transmitting and receiving transducers are mounted side by side with a lens in front. This lens makes the transmitted beam overlap the region where the receiving transducer is sensitive.

Consider a volume element of blood so small that the velocity profile is essentially constant inside it. The velocity of the element is v and the angle between the ultrasonic beam and the velocity vector is θ as illustrated in Figure 3.2. The Doppler shift in frequency of the backscattered sound is then

$$f_d = 2f_0 \frac{v\cos\theta}{c} \tag{3.5}$$

We see that the velocity component (see Figure 2.4) along the ultrasonic beam, *the radial velocity,* produces the Doppler shift. f_0 is the transmitted ultrasonic frequency, and $c \approx 1560$ m/s is the velocity of sound in blood.

The Doppler shift as a function of radial velocity is shown in Figure 3.3 for $f_0 = 1, 2,$ and 5 MHz. The Doppler shift is proportional to the radial velocity and the transmitted ultrasonic frequency.

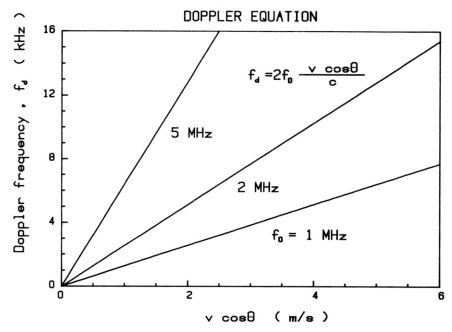

Fig. 3–3. **Doppler equation.**

With a continuous wave instrument we observe all blood motion along the beam, i.e., there is *no range resolution.* Since the different blood elements have different velocities, a spectrum of Doppler-shifted frequencies is received.

B. Pulsed Wave (PW) Doppler Technique

By pulsing the ultrasonic beam, one can obtain range resolution along the beam. A short burst of ultrasound is transmitted with a repetition frequency (f_s). The backscattered signal is received with the same transducer and sampled with a time delay (T_d) after the pulse transmission. Thus, we select the signal from scatterers in a range cell at a depth

$$z = \frac{cT_d}{2} \tag{3.6}$$

The length of the range cell along the beam is determined by the length of the transmitted pulse, and the transverse dimensions are determined by the beam width. For PEDOF,* the instrument we have used, the diameter of the

*Vingmed a/s, Oslo, Norway

range cell is ≈ 7 mm and its length is ≈ 7 mm. These are approximate values since the boundaries of the beam are diffuse (see Figure 3.1) and the transmitted burst has slow rise and fall times. Therefore, neither the transverse nor the longitudinal boundaries of the range cell are sharp.

In the PW technique we sample the Doppler signal once for each pulse transmission. The reconstruction of the continuous Doppler signal from these discrete samples introduces an ambiguity, as illustrated in Figure 3.4.

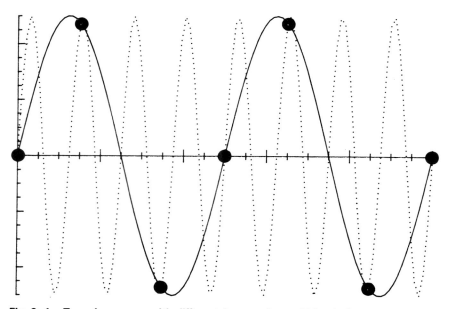

Fig. 3–4.   Two sine waves with different frequencies and identical samples.

Here, two sine waves that have different frequencies pass through the same samples. If we know that

$$|f_d| < \frac{1}{2} f_s \qquad\qquad (3.7)$$

we can select the signal with the lowest frequency and thus obtain uniqueness. If $|f_d| > \frac{1}{2} f_s$, a phenomenon called *frequency aliasing* will cause ambiguity in determining the Doppler shift. This is discussed in more detail in Sections 3.6 and 8.4C.

To avoid ambiguity in depth, one must sample the backscattered signal before the next pulse is transmitted. To measure at higher depths, one must lower the pulse repetition frequency, f_s, and thereby lower the maximum

Doppler shift that can be detected (Equation 3.7). Since the Doppler shift is proportional to the radial velocity of the scatterer, we obtain the following limit on the range velocity product

$$\mathbf{v_m R} = \frac{\mathbf{c}^2}{\mathbf{8f_0}} \tag{3.8}$$

where v_m is the absolute value of the maximum radial velocity that can be measured at a depth (R).

v_m as a function of R is shown in Figure 3.5 for f_0 = 1, 2, and 5 MHz. For a fixed depth, R, the maximum velocity that can be measured is inversely proportional to the ultrasonic frequency. We thus see that at 7 cm depth we can measure velocities up to .87m/s for f_0 = 5 MHz, 2.17m/s for f_0 = 2 MHz, and 4.34m/s for f_0 = 1 MHz. Owing to practical limitations in the instrument filters, these values are reduced by a factor of .9.

The resolution, however, is reduced when the ultrasonic frequency is reduced. For practical reasons, we have chosen f_0 = 2 MHz in the instrument. Two pulse repetition frequencies are used. In the high repetition rate we can measure velocities up to 1.7 m/s between 2 and 8 cm depth and 1.1 m/s between 8 and 12 cm depth. When velocities above these limits are present, the instrument can be switched to the CW mode where range

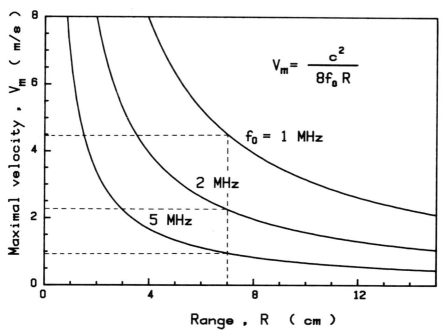

Fig. 3–5.   Range velocity product.

resolution is lost, but where there is no limit on the maximum velocity that can be measured. Usually such high velocities are found in localized regions only, so that range resolution is not necessary to quantitate the high velocity. Localization of the disturbed flow within the heart can be done with the PW mode. It is therefore practical to have a combined instrument where one can switch between the CW and PW modes.

The limit on the maximum measurable velocity is caused by the sampling theorem (Equation 3.7). To avoid range ambiguity, we cannot have more than one pulse traveling in the heart at the same time. This situation is illustrated in Figure 3.6. This limits the pulse repetition frequency (f_s).

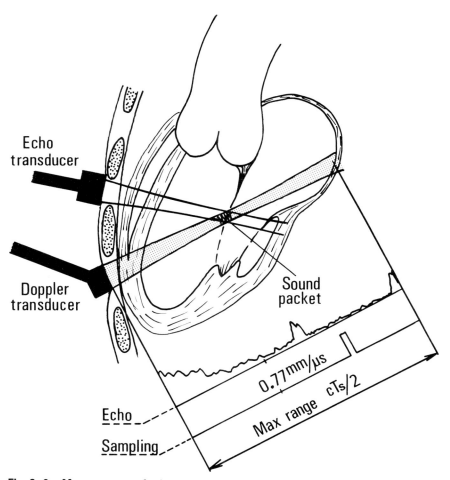

Fig. 3–6. Measurement of mitral blood velocity without range ambiguity.

If we increase f_s, we can measure higher Doppler shifts. However, if f_s is increased so much that several pulses are in the heart at the same time, there is a problem with range ambiguity, as illustrated in Figure 3.7. Here, echoes from both the left ventricle and the left atrium at the same time might cause confusion. However, both in normal individuals and in those with mitral stenosis, the velocities in the left ventricle are higher than those in the left atrium. The range ambiguity can be resolved if we are interested in the highest velocities only.

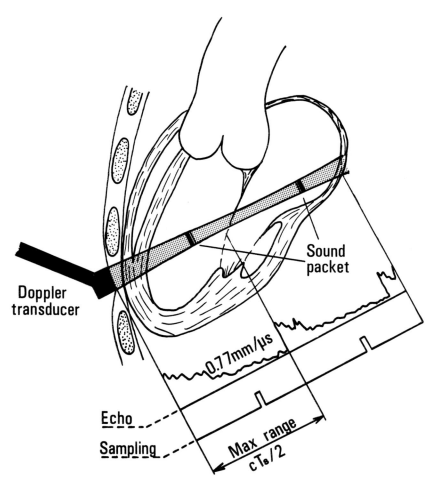

Fig. 3–7.   Measurement of the mitral blood velocity with a pulse repetition frequency so high that range ambiguity might cause a problem.

With combined mitral stenosis and regurgitation, there are high velocities in the left ventricle toward the transducer in diastole, and high velocities in the left atrium which move away from the transducer in systole, resolving the range ambiguity in this situation.

One situation that causes a problem is dynamic left ventricular obstruction with mitral regurgitation, which shows high velocities away from the transducer in systole, in both the left ventricle and left atrium. Since the regurgitant velocity usually is the highest, the ventricular velocity can be obscured by the atrial velocity.

From the previous discussion we see that it is possible to measure higher velocities in the pulsed mode than by Equation 3.8, if we allow range ambiguity to occur. In a sense, CW can be thought of as the limit of increasing the pulse repetition to infinity, and the range resolution is completely ambiguous. If one knows the anatomy, the problem of range ambiguity can often be resolved as described. With the instrument used, there are two pulse repetition frequencies: one that gives a maximum depth of 8 cm and one that gives a maximum depth of 12 cm. When the instrument is adjusted to 3 cm in the short range mode, we may also observe ambiguous echoes from the former pulse at $8 + 3 = 11$ cm depth.

Using complex spectral analysis, we can measure Doppler shifts above $\frac{1}{2} f_s$. If we have only one sign (positive or negative) of the Doppler shift, we can detect Doppler shifts up to f_s. This is discussed in Sections 3.6 and 8.4C.

3.4 RELATIONSHIP BETWEEN VELOCITY PROFILE AND DOPPLER SIGNAL

A. Relationship Between Velocity Profile and Signal Spectrum

Since the different volume elements of the blood have different velocities, the signal is composed of a spectrum of Doppler-shifted frequencies. The intensity distribution gives an indication of the velocity distribution inside the observed region of blood. We shall discuss this in more detail.

First, the *velocity distribution* is not the same as the velocity profile. The latter gives the velocity as a function of position in the cross section and can, for instance, take the form of a parabola (see Figure 2.6). The velocity distribution, $f(v)$, gives the amount of blood flowing with a certain velocity, v. A parabolic velocity profile gives a rectangular velocity distribution over the cross section, as shown in Figure 3.8a. With a beam so wide that all points in the cross section are observed equally well, the *power spectrum* of the Doppler signal from this velocity distribution appears as shown in Figure 3.8b. The power spectrum $G(f)$ is defined as

$$G(f)\, df = \begin{cases} \textbf{Average amount of power of the signal} \\ \textbf{in the frequency range (f, f + df)} \end{cases}$$

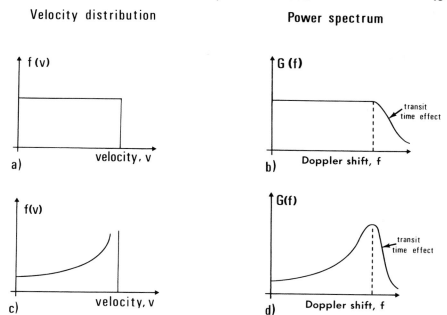

Velocity distribution   **Power spectrum**

Fig. 3–8. Velocity distribution and signal power spectrum using wide beam for parabolic profile (a and b) and a blunt profile (c and d).

We note that the spectrum is rounded at the upper part due to the transit time effect. The reason for this is that the received signal from each scatterer is of finite duration in time, since the element moves through the ultrasonic beam. Because a sharp frequency can only be obtained if the signal is of infinite duration in time, in this case we obtain a frequency line centered around f_d and with a line width, Δf,

$$\frac{\Delta f}{f_d} = \frac{\lambda}{2L\cos\theta} \qquad (3.9)$$

where L is the traversed length of the scatterer through the beam. This is illustrated in Figure 3.9 and discussed in more detail in Section 8.2A.

If $L\cos\theta > 5\lambda$, which is most often the case, the relative transit time broadening is less than 10%, which is negligible.

Figure 3.8c shows the velocity distribution for a profile that is more flat than the parabolic. There is more blood flowing with high velocities, increasing the spectral intensity near the maximum value as in Figure 3.8d. The form of the Doppler spectrum is, therefore, influenced by the velocity profile.

The different spectra produce different characteristics of the audible sound of the Doppler signal. The wide spectrum in Figure 3.8b produces a harsh

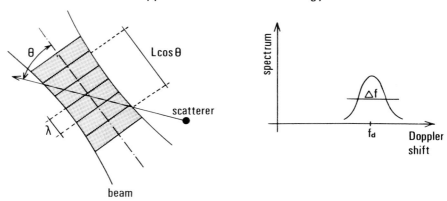

Fig. 3–9. Transit time effect.

sound, whereas the narrow-band spectrum in Figure 3.8d produces a more whistling sound.

However, the range cell often does not cover the artery completely. *What we observe is the velocity distribution within the range cell, and not within the whole artery lumen.* In addition, because of the varying intensity of the beam (see Section 3.1), we observe a weighted form of the velocity distribution, the weighing being performed by the varying intensity of the ultrasonic beam. *Therefore, the deduction of the velocity profile from the spectrum is not unique, although the spectrum can give an indication of the form of the profile as is demonstrated in the next section.*

B.   Time-Variable Velocity Fields

The Doppler signal has a random (stochastic) nature since the relative location of the scattering red cells is random. To obtain an exact estimate of the signal power spectrum, this estimate should be taken over infinite time. Because the blood velocity changes with time, however, we must estimate the spectrum over such a short time interval that the velocity can be considered essentially constant (~10 ms). This leaves errors in the estimate, which is schematically illustrated in Figure 3.10. This random uncertainty also complicates the deduction of the velocity profile from the spectrum.

Since the velocity varies with time, we obtain a time-variable spectrum. This is illustrated in Figure 3.11, which shows a three-dimensional plot of the spectrum as a function of time. Perhaps a more illustrative way to display the spectrum is as the grey-scale plot shown in Figure 3.12. Time is along the horizontal axes, while frequency is along the vertical axes. The grey scale indicates the amplitude of the spectrum.

The spectrum analyzer used operates in discrete time and frequency. This causes the discrete nature of the grey-scale plot. The stochastic nature of the spectrum estimate is found as random variations in the grey scale.

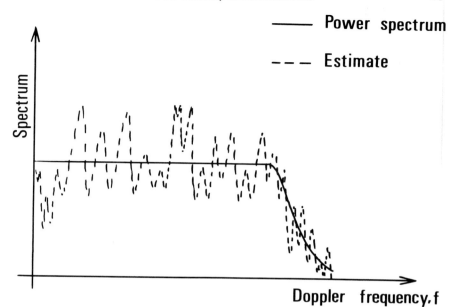

Fig. 3–10.   Stochastic uncertainty in spectral estimate.

The width of each frequency line, $\triangle f$, in Figure 3.12 is inversely proportional to the length in time, T, of the part of the signal used to compute the spectrum

$$\triangle f = \frac{1}{T} \tag{3.10}$$

Thus, the area of the time-frequency cells in Figure 3.12 is unity ($\triangle f \cdot T = 1$). The spectrum analyzer has 64 frequencies. For a data time, T = 7.5 ms, the analyzer covers a range of

$$64\triangle f = 8.5 \text{ kHz} \tag{3.11}$$

which corresponds to ±1.7 m/s for 2 MHz ultrasound.

The spectrum analyzer has four different amplitude compression characteristics for the grey-scale display. These are shown in Figure 3.13. The effect on the grey-scale plot of the different characteristics is shown in Figure 3.14.

The spectra shown in Figure 3.14 are from measurements in the right common carotid artery. A wide beam is used so that the artery lumen is approximately evenly insonified. The band width of the spectrum is much narrower in systole than in diastole because the velocity profile is flatter in

Power

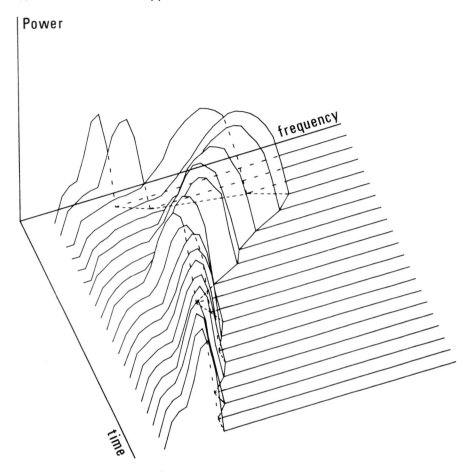

Fig. 3–11.   Three-dimensional plot of time-variable spectrum.

systole than in diastole, in accordance with the discussion in Section 2.3A. We also have some negative Doppler shifts in the early deceleration phase in the late systole. This is probably caused by the reversal of the velocity profile near the walls, due to the retardation, as shown in Figure 2.7b.

3.5   SIMPLIFIED FORMS OF SPECTRAL ANALYSIS

Complete spectral analysis of the Doppler signal gives all information available in the signal. Although the electronics for performing such analysis have become quite simple, the equipment for grey-scale display of the spectrum is still expensive.

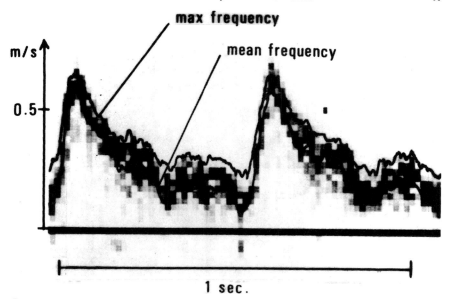

Fig. 3–12. Grey-scale plot of the Doppler spectrum together with mean and maximum frequency trace.

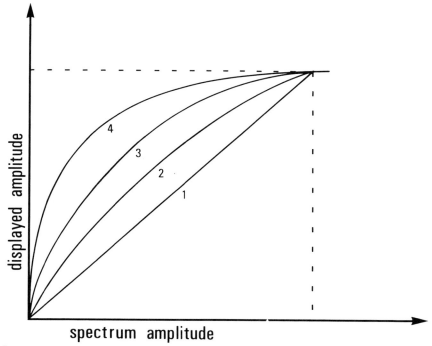

Fig. 3–13. Grey-scale amplitude compression curves of spectrum analyzer.

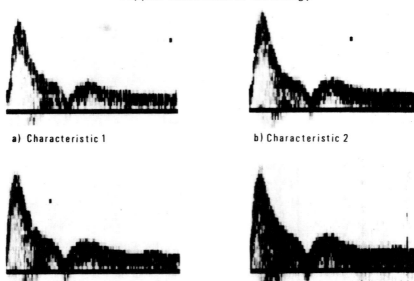

a) Characteristic 1   b) Characteristic 2

c) Characteristic 3   d) Characteristic 4

Fig. 3–14.   Effect of compression on the grey-scale display of the spectrum.

A number of single-frequency estimators, using single time-variable voltages, have, therefore, been developed. These can be recorded on signal recorders (like ECG recorders) already existing in most laboratories. The estimators can give the maximum frequency,[2,3] the mean frequency,[4-6] and the root mean square (rms) frequency (zero crosser)[7,8] of the spectrum. The relationship between the spectrum and the maximum and mean frequencies is indicated in Figure 3.12. The rms frequency lies somewhere between the maximum and the mean frequencies.

The maximum frequency has proved to be valuable in diagnosis and assessment of heart lesions (see Chapter 5). This can be obtained from a maximum frequency estimator or from the spectrum. The time-interval histogram is another method of analysis that has been used.[9] This gives the mean frequency of the spectrum and an indication of the spectrum width,[10,11] but not the detailed form of the spectrum. It does not give the maximum frequency either.

A.   Estimation of Maximum Frequency

One problem in estimating the maximum frequency is the lack of any sharp definition of it. The spectrum falls off slowly due to transit time effects and stochastic uncertainty in the spectral estimate. In addition, the signal contains noise, as indicated in Figure 3.15. The true maximum frequency in the signal is therefore determined by the noise.

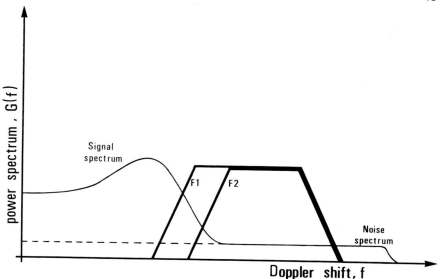

Fig. 3–15. **Principle of maximum frequency estimation.**

We have used an ad hoc definition of the maximum frequency using the two frequency windows shown in Figure 3.15. The relative position between the windows is fixed, but they can be moved together along the frequency axis. The powers in the two windows are equated so that

$$\frac{P_2}{P_1} = \alpha \qquad\qquad (3.12)$$

where α is a small number ($\approx .1$). P_1 is the signal power in frequency window F_1 and P_2 is the power in frequency window F_2. Equation 3.12 can be satisfied only when the lower slope of F_2 is located at a falling edge in the spectrum. If P_2/P_1 is less than α, the position of the windows is moved to the left, and if P_2/P_1 is greater than α, the position of the windows is moved to the right. Hence, an edge in the spectrum can be tracked.

The ability of the estimator to track an edge in the spectrum depends on both the slope of the edge and its amplitude above the noise. When the velocity increases in the jet in a valve stenosis, the spectral intensity corresponding to the high velocities decreases. We then can have an intensity distribution in the spectrum as indicated in Figure 3.16. It can be difficult to track the maximum frequency of such a spectrum. For optimal results the level of the signal before it enters the estimator should be adjusted so that the estimator is barely tracking the maximum signal frequency, to avoid the possibility of the estimator locking on the noise. In PEDOF a lamp lights when a sufficient signal level at the estimator input is reached. One should

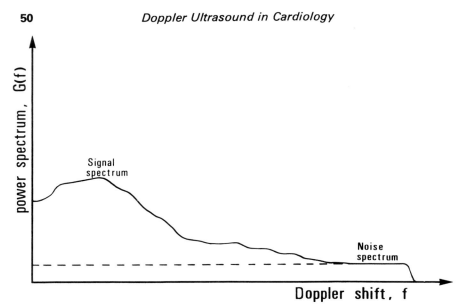

Fig. 3–16. **Spectrum where it is difficult to estimate the maximum frequency.**

start with a low value of the gain and then increase it so that the lamp is lit. This produces a curve similar to the one in Figure 3.17a which shows measurements of an aortic stenosis. If the gain is adjusted too high, the noise starts to influence the measurement, and a curve similar to the one in Figure 3.17b may be obtained. *To be sure that the estimator is producing correct results, one can check that the estimator output is independent of some increasing input gain adjustment after the lamp has lit, and before the output takes off on the noise.*

B.   Estimation of Mean Frequency

The mean frequency of the spectrum is the weighted average Doppler shift for each instant of time. It can therefore *vary with time as illustrated in Figure 3.12.* The mean Doppler shift is interesting because the artery, if uniformly insonified, will be proportional to the space-average velocity in the artery (see Sections 2.1, 2.2A). There are a couple of obstacles to this, however. The mean Doppler shift is proportional to a weighted mean of the velocity distribution in the observed region, the weighting being caused by the variation in the field intensity from the transducer. If the beam is so wide that there is uniform insonification of the artery, this mean Doppler shift will be approximately proportional to the space-average velocity in the artery. It is, however, hard to control whether one has uniform insonification or not.

To remove signals from tissue, one uses a high-pass filter. This also removes the signals from slowly moving blood. This leads to an overestimation

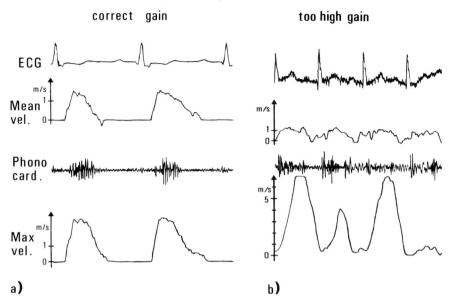

Fig. 3–17. a) Correct adjustment of maximum frequency estimator. b) Too high input gain on the estimator. Measurements on aortic stenosis.

of the mean velocity. The degree of overestimation depends on the relative amount of slowly moving blood, i.e., the form of the velocity profile. The effect of this on the estimator output is shown in Figure 3.18.[12]

3.6   CLINICAL SIGNIFICANCE OF VELOCITY AMBIGUITY IN PW MODE

In Section 3.3 we discussed how the maximum measurable velocity is limited in the PW mode. This section covers the clinical significance of this.

Figure 3.19 shows how a typical Doppler spectrum is distorted when velocity ambiguity occurs. The left panel shows the spectrum with unambiguous measurements (CW mode). When the pulsed mode is used, ambiguity cuts the spectrum off at $\frac{1}{2}f_s$ and moves the top down $-f_s$ as illustrated. This shift of the frequency spectrum is termed *frequency aliasing*. The mean frequency estimator calculates the average of both the positive and the negative (ambiguous) parts of the spectrum. Thus, there is a dip in the mean frequency output as illustrated. The maximum frequency flattens off at $\frac{1}{2}f_s$.

Figure 3.20 illustrates how this effect is observed in the clinical situation. The figure shows measurements of an aortic stenosis. The left panel shows measurements in the PW mode. The mean velocity first goes positive before

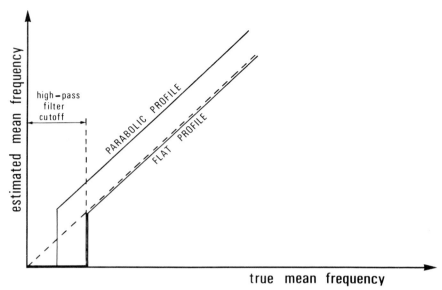

Fig. 3–18.   Offset of mean frequency estimator due to high-pass filters.

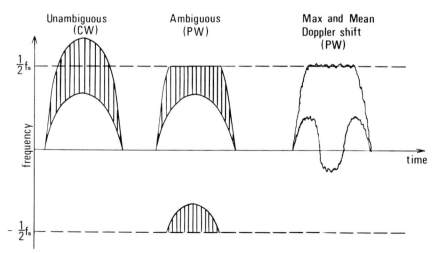

Fig. 3–19.   Frequency aliasing causing ambiguity in the Doppler spectrum in the PW mode.

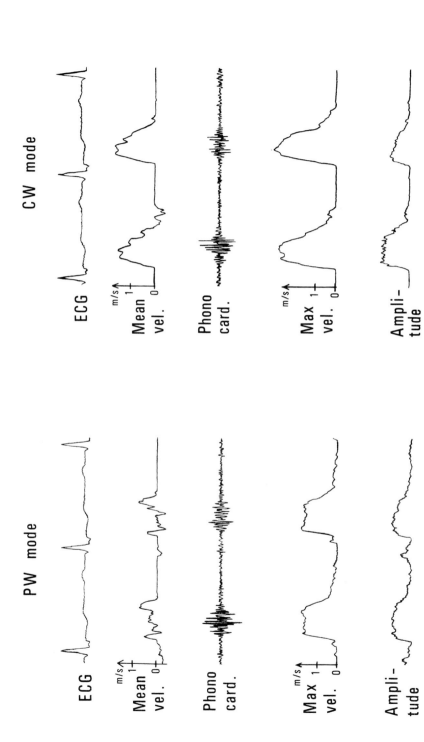

Fig. 3–20.   Frequency aliasing in a clinical situation. Aortic stenosis measured from the second right intercostal space.

53

a negative dip and then positive again, as in Figure 3.19. The maximum velocity flattens off at about 1.7 m/s, which is the instrument's limit. When we switch to the CW mode, the correct reproduction of both mean and maximum velocity is given.

The same effect is also observed in Figure 5.10 for mitral stenosis and Figure 5.23 for infundibular pulmonary stenosis. In the latter the frequency aliasing occurs at a depth of 6 cm. We see from the amplitude of the Doppler signal that this is located below the valve, which means that the obstruction is subvalvular. If one switches the instrument to the CW mode, a peak velocity of 2.5 m/s is found, which gives a pressure drop of 25 mm Hg across the obstruction (see Section 2.4A).

When the Doppler frequency exceeds $\frac{1}{2}f_s$, f_s is subtracted from the frequency. In this way a negative frequency is obtained. This is similar to the stroboscope effect observed in movies. A movie is also a sampled system, usually running at 30 samples (images) per second. When the motion is slow, the eye, which functions as a low-pass filter, reconstructs the motion. If the motion is too fast (e.g., the wheel on a cart in a Western movie), the wheel starts spinning backwards. This is because the sample theorem is violated. If the frequency increases more, it will flip over to negative frequencies every time the apparent frequency passes $\frac{1}{2}f_s$. This is illustrated in Figure 3.21.

Figure 3.22 shows the effect of aliasing when the velocity limit is heavily exceeded. Even though there are only positive Doppler shifts, frequency

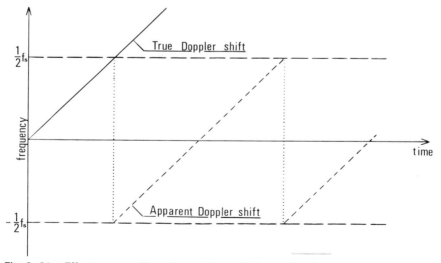

Fig. 3–21. Effect on sampling of a continuously increasing Doppler frequency.

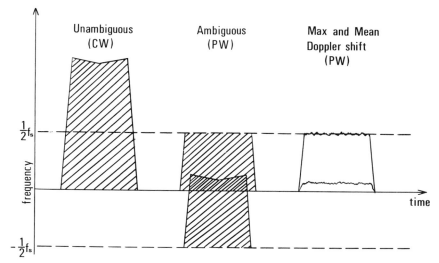

Fig. 3–22.   Severe frequency aliasing in PW mode.

aliasing in the pulsed mode makes it look as if we have both positive and negative Doppler shifts in equal amounts.

The aliasing phenomenon has often caused confusion in the literature when one is measuring high velocities with a pulsed instrument. High velocities have been observed as equal amounts of positive and negative velocities, which in turn have been diagnosed as turbulence.

Figure 3.19 demonstrates that one can reconstruct the true spectrum from the ambiguous spectrum by taking the lower part and putting it on the top of $\frac{1}{2}f_s$. This way we can study Doppler shifts up to

$$f_d < \frac{1}{2}f_s + \frac{1}{2}f_s = f_s \qquad \textbf{(3.13)}$$

i.e., twice the limit of the sampling theorem (Equation 3.7). This requires that we have only positive Doppler shifts. If we have some negative Doppler shifts at the same time, we cannot measure Doppler shifts up to f_s. In general, using this technique, we can measure Doppler shifts in the range of

$$-\frac{1}{2}f_s + \triangle < f_d < \frac{1}{2}f_s + \triangle \qquad \textbf{(3.14)}$$

where $\triangle$ can be chosen arbitrarily. If $\triangle = -\frac{1}{2}f_s$, we obtain

$$-f_s < f_d < 0 \qquad \textbf{(3.15)}$$

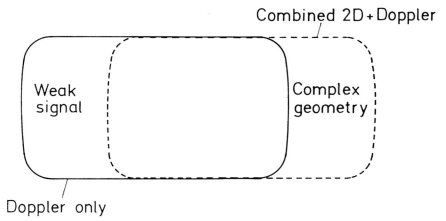

Combined 2D + Doppler

Weak
signal

Complex
geometry

Doppler only

Fig. 3–23. Venn diagram illustrating the group of patients who can be diagnosed with a single Doppler only and a combined 2D + Doppler system. The areas do not give quantitative information about the size of the groups.

and if $\triangle = \dfrac{1}{2}f_s$, we obtain

$$0 < f_d < f_s \qquad\qquad\qquad (3.16)$$

Thus, if we have only one sign of the Doppler shift, we can measure velocities up to twice the limit given in Equation 3.8. The spectrum analyzer that we have used* has the necessary features to measure velocities up to 3.57 m/s at 8 cm depth. If we use Equation 2.2, this equals a pressure drop across a stenotic valve of 50 mm Hg.

3.7 COMBINATION BETWEEN ULTRASONIC DOPPLER AND AMPLITUDE IMAGING SYSTEMS

The optimization of an ultrasonic pulse Doppler velocity measurement system and the optimization of an ultrasonic pulse echo amplitude imaging system are subject to somewhat different concerns (see Appendix B). Combining a pulse Doppler and M-mode imaging system leads to trade-offs between the optimal design of the two systems. Moreover, for M-mode examination, the transducer should be angled from different directions than for Doppler examinations. This is illustrated for mitral valve examination in Figure 3.6.

We have also found that the combination with M-mode does not provide good guidance for the Doppler beam. The Doppler signal itself can be used equally well for location purposes, as will be discussed in Chapter 4. Two-

*Daisy, Vingmed a/s, Oslo, Norway

dimensional images give a better guidance for the Doppler measurement than the M-mode. This is especially useful where one has complex geometry, as in complex congenital heart defects. However, existing systems suffer from the trade-offs between Doppler and image optimization, which reduces the quality of the Doppler measurement.

A specially optimized Doppler system is able to detect weaker signals. As indicated in Figure 3.23, in many patients equal results may be obtained with either separate or combined Doppler plus 2D systems. In some, a combined Doppler plus 2D is better with a more rapid and unambiguous localization of the range cell. In other patients, especially those with weak signals, separate systems give better results. *We should also bear in mind that a continuous-wave Doppler is often necessary to quantitate high velocities.*

REFERENCES

1. Angelsen B.A.J.: A theoretical study of the scattering of ultrasound from blood. IEEE Trans. Biomed. Eng. 1980; BME-27: 61-67.
2. Angelsen B.A.J.: Analog estimation of the maximum frequency of Doppler spectra in ultrasonic blood velocity measurements. Report 76-21-W, Division of Engineering Cybernetics, The Norwegian Institute of Technology, Trondheim 1976.
3. Brubakk A.O., Angelsen B.A.J., Hatle L.: Diagnosis of valvular heart disease. Cardiovasc. Res. 1977; 11: 461-469.
4. Arts M.G.J., Roevros J.M.J.G.: On the instantaneous measurement of blood flow by ultrasonic means. Med. Biol. Eng. 1972; 10: 23-34.
5. Pawula R.F.: Analysis of center frequency of a power spectrum. IEEE Trans. Inf. Theory 1968; IT-14: 669-675.
6. Angelsen B.A.J., Brubakk A.O.: Transcutaneous measurement of blood flow velocity in the human aorta. Cardiovasc. Res. 1976; 10: 368-379.
7. Reneman R.S., Clarke H.F., Simmons N., Spencer M.P.: In vivo comparison of electromagnetic and Doppler flowmeters: With special attention to the processing of analog Doppler flow signal. Cardiovasc. Res. 1973; 7: 557-566.
8. Papoulis A.: Probability, Random Variables and Stochastic Processes. Tokyo, McGraw-Hill Book Co. 1965: 487.
9. Baker D.W., Rubenstein G.A., Lorch G.S.: Pulsed Doppler echocardiography: Principles and applications. Am. J. Med. 1977; 63: 69-80.
10. Angelsen B.A.J.: Spectral estimation of a narrow-band Gaussian process from the distribution of the distance between adjacent zeros. IEEE Trans. Biomed. Eng. 1980; BME-27: 108-110.
11. Burckhardt C.B.: Comparison between spectrum and time interval histogram of ultrasound Doppler signals. Ultrasound Med. Biol. 1981; 7: 79-82.
12. Gill R.W.: Performance of the mean frequency Doppler modulator. Ultrasound Med. Biol. 1979; 5: 237-247.

4

Pulsed Doppler Recording of Intracardiac Blood Flow Velocities: Orientation and Normal Velocity Patterns

4.1 INTRODUCTION

In cardiac diagnosis Doppler ultrasound has mainly been used in the pulsed mode (PW) to record velocity patterns in the heart. M-mode[1,2] or, more recently, two-dimensional (2D) echocardiography[3,4] has been used for localization of the region of the Doppler recording. Doppler ultrasound alone has been used to record blood flow velocities in the descending or ascending aorta with continuous wave (CW) Doppler[5-8] or with pulsed and CW Doppler.[9,10] Blood flow velocities within the heart have also been recorded noninvasively without the aid of simultaneous echocardiography with CW Doppler[11] and with a combined CW and pulsed Doppler.[12] The use of Doppler to record valve movements within the heart was described earlier.[13]

Doppler signals from blood flow velocities are best recorded with the ultrasound beam aligned to the velocity while optimal echocardiograms are obtained with the beam at a right angle to the structure recorded. Optimal Doppler signals are therefore obtained from other positions and angles than the usual M-mode echocardiogram. Good Doppler signals are often easier to find using the Doppler signal itself as a guide instead of the echocardiogram. Continuous wave Doppler can be used to find the characteristic velocity patterns in the various parts of the heart. Changing to pulsed Doppler allows the various flow velocity signals to be located in depth. The sound of valve movements differs clearly from that of blood flow. The valve movements can, therefore, be used for orientation as landmarks within the heart in much the same way as in M-mode echocardiography. The following section describes how the valve movements, together with the velocity curves from blood flow, make orientation within the heart possible with Doppler ultrasound alone, and how this approach facilitates optimal

Doppler recordings. Velocity curves from various parts of the heart in normal individuals are presented.

4.2 METHOD AND APPLICATION

A combined pulsed and continuous wave Doppler is used (see Section 3.3). The ultrasonic frequency is 2 MHz. The instrument has a nondirectional maximum frequency estimator, and a directional mean frequency estimator which also gives the direction of flow (positive with flow towards the transducer and negative when away from the transducer) (see Sections 3.4, 3.5, and 3.6). The amplitude of the Doppler signal is recorded separately. The valve movements give strong reflections and are heard as loud clicks while the sound of blood flow is more continuous and less intense. The valve movements show up, therefore, as spikes in the amplitude of the Doppler signal, as shown in Figure 4.2. Since the velocity of the valves is comparable to that of the blood, the valve movements are not as clearly indicated in the velocity tracings. The amplitude of the Doppler signal is useful, therefore, for timing of the valve movements as well as for localization of the range cell close to or within a valve area.

For a signal to pass through the instrument's high-pass filter, a certain velocity is required. A cut-off frequency of 500 Hz is most often used. In the presence of low velocities of valve movements or of blood flow, a lower-frequency filter is used. When high velocities are present, a higher frequency filter can be better. Mean and maximal velocity and amplitude of Doppler signal are recorded together with ECG and phonocardiogram on an ordinary paper recorder.*

To calculate the velocity of blood flow, both the Doppler frequency shift from the velocity and the angle between velocity and ultrasound beam are necessary. The Doppler equation describes the relation between frequency shift (f_2), maximal velocity (v), and angle (θ) between ultrasound beam and velocity:

$$f_2 = \frac{2 \cdot f_0 \cdot v \cdot \cos \theta}{c} \tag{4.1}$$

where f_0 is the transmitted frequency and c is the velocity of sound in blood. With an angle of zero, the velocity is obtained from the frequency shift alone. The higher the velocity, the larger the frequency shift. It increases when the angle to the velocity decreases. It is highest when ultrasound beam and velocity are aligned. The audio signal then contains the highest frequency sounds.

Since one cannot at present determine angles to velocities within the heart, one can instead use the frequency shift of the Doppler signal to try to

---

*Elema Mingograph

obtain a small enough angle to the velocity so the angle can be neglected in the Doppler equation. With small angles (20 to 25°), underestimation of velocity by neglecting the angle in the calculation is small (6% at 20°).

CW Doppler is used to detect where Doppler signals from the various parts of the heart can be obtained, and to detect the position and angle where the highest frequency shifts from the blood flow are found. For each velocity pattern, pulsed Doppler is then used to localize it in distance from the transducer and in relation to the valves. The pulsed mode is also used to record the magnitude of the various velocities provided these are within the limit for the pulsed mode. With maximal velocities above this limit, the continuous mode is used.

Since valve movements give stronger signals, these are recorded over a larger area than the weaker signals from blood flow. They may therefore be recorded even when located a little outside the sample volume, probably due to side lobes in the beam (see Section 3.1) and to reverberations.

4.3 CLINICAL EXAMINATION

A. Flow Velocity Curves in the Left Ventricle

The examination starts by locating the mitral or tricuspid valve movements. To record velocity of mitral flow, one places the transducer at or slightly medial to the apex and directs it backward, slightly medial and upward. The CW mode is used for rapid localization of flow signals, and the transducer is then moved and angled until the highest frequency shifts are obtained (i.e, the direction with the smallest angle to the velocity of flow). The pulsed mode is then used to record the velocities in various depths along this beam direction.

Figure 4.1 (3) shows an example of a normal velocity curve from the inflow part of the left ventricle (mitral flow). In sinus rhythm this consists of two peaks: The first is the velocity of early diastolic filling, and the second one, usually smaller, represents increase in velocity following atrial contraction. In atrial fibrillation the second peak is missing and in other atrial arrhythmias several peaks may be seen, one at each atrial contraction. When the transducer is angled a little more medially and superiorly, velocity of mitral flow in diastole is still recorded; in addition, however, flow away from the transducer is recorded as shown in Figure 4.1 (2) (i.e., both left ventricular inflow and outflow are present in the sample volume). When the transducer is directed still more medially and superiorly, only flow away from the transducer in systole is recorded (1). In this way the inflow and middle and outflow regions of the left ventricle are located. The lower part of Figure 4.1 shows a scan from the outflow to the inflow region of the left ventricle. For further localization within the left ventricle, the depth where the valve movements can be recorded is noted.

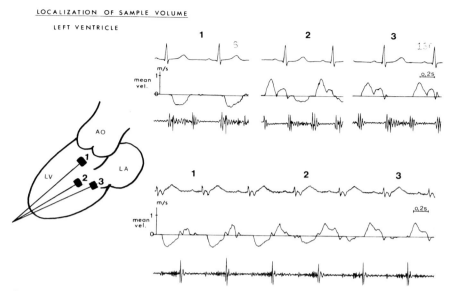

Fig. 4–1. Flow velocity patterns in the left ventricle recorded with pulsed Doppler. In the outflow region close to the aortic valve (1), only velocity of systolic flow away from the transducer (negative) toward the aorta is recorded. Lower down in the left ventricle or when angling the transducer more toward the mitral valve (2), both flow velocity away from the transducer in systole and velocity of mitral flow toward the transducer in diastole are recorded. When the transducer is directed more toward the mitral valve, only flow velocity toward the transducer in diastole is found. This consists of two peaks in sinus rhythm: one represents early diastolic filling, the second represents increase in velocity following atrial contraction. The lower curve shows a scan from the outflow to the inflow region of the left ventricle. AO—aorta; LA—left atrium; LV—left ventricle.

Figure 4.2 shows recording with pulsed Doppler at various depths towards the mitral valve. With the sample volume in the left ventricle below the mitral valve, only the velocity of blood flow is recorded. When the sample volume is moved deeper, the opening movement of the mitral valve is also heard as a short snapping sound preceding the flow velocity signal in early diastole. In the recording, the valve movement is best shown in the amplitude curve. If the sample volume is moved further back 1 to 2 cm or more, depending on the size and movement of the mitral valve, the closing movement of the valve at the end of diastole is also heard. Further back, at the mitral orifice, the opening movement is no longer heard, the velocity of forward diastolic flow is decreasing, but the valve closure is clearly recorded. At this level, velocity following atrial contraction may be better recorded than the velocity in early diastole.

In the left atrium, velocity of forward flow is not usually recorded, but behind the left atrium velocity of flow towards the transducer in systole is

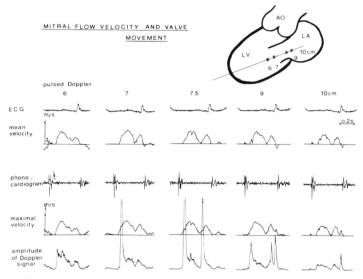

Fig. 4–2. Pulsed Doppler recording of mitral flow velocity. The sample volume is moved stepwise toward the valve. The mean (directional) and maximal velocity curves (nondirectional) change little. At 6 cm increase in velocity following atrial contraction is less well recorded than closer to the valve. The amplitude curve shows the valve movements better separated from flow velocity. At 6 cm valve movements are not recorded, at 7 cm the valve opening is clearly heard and recorded, and at 7.5 cm also the valve reopens following atrial contraction. At 9 cm the opening movements are less prominent, but mitral valve closure is present. At 10 cm only valve closure is recorded and flow velocity is reduced.

sometimes recorded, most likely from flow in the descending aorta. In some patients the mid-diastolic closing movement of the mitral valve is also heard as well as the reopening of the valve prior to flow velocity following atrial contraction. With high cardiac output as well as other conditions with increased flow across the valve (e.g., shunts, mitral regurgitation), the diastolic flutter of the mitral valve during peak velocity is easily heard as frequent, repeated valve movements. This valve flutter is clearly different from the continuous valve flutter throughout diastole heard in aortic regurgitation. With restricted valve movements, as in severe left ventricular hypertrophy without dilatation, the mitral valve movements are recorded over a much smaller area than normal; conversely, with enlarged valve cusps, as in mitral valve prolapse, they are recorded over a larger area than usual.

B. Aortic Valve Area

When the sample volume is placed in the left ventricular outflow tract and moved up toward the aortic valve area, the aortic valve closure is first recorded in addition to the flow velocity (Figure 4.3). If the sample volume is moved to 1 to 1.5 cm further up toward the aorta, the opening movement of the valve is also recorded. At this level a slight change in the velocity curve is usually observed with a slight increase in velocity and earlier peak velocity than below the valve. This level may, therefore, represent the valve orifice with the transition from a left ventricular to an aortic flow velocity curve. When the sample volume is moved further up, the closing movement of the aortic valve is first lost, then the valve opening.

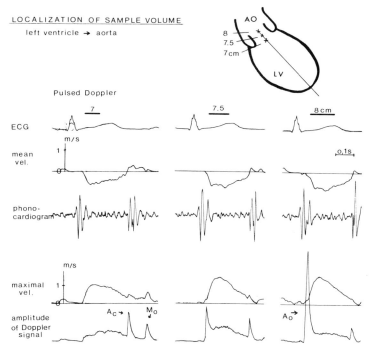

Fig. 4–3. When one is moving the sample volume upward in the left ventricular outflow tract, the closing movement of the aortic valve (Ac) is first noted (7 cm). With a small left ventricle, the mitral valve opening (Mo) may be recorded at the same time. At 7.5 cm aortic valve opening(Ao) and closure are equally well recorded. A slight increase in velocity is found at this level, and the velocity curve becomes similar to that recorded in the ascending aorta above valve level. When one is moving the sample volume upward (8 cm), aortic valve opening is better and closure is less clearly recorded.

C.   Flow Velocity Curves in the Right Ventricle

Velocity of flow through the tricuspid valve is usually recorded from the same position as above, but with the ultrasonic beam directed more forward and to the right. Apart from the different location, tricuspid flow velocity can be distinguished from mitral by a lower velocity and by the variation in the velocity with respiration. Figure 4.4 shows examples of mitral and tricuspid flow velocity from normal subjects. With inspiration, velocity of tricuspid flow increases and can be recorded throughout diastole. This change in the Doppler signal with respiration is usually easy to hear. Velocity of flow through the tricuspid valve may also be recorded from the third, fourth, or fifth intercostal spaces at the left sternal border or from the subcostal position, but the angle between ultrasound beam and velocity may be too large in the latter position to obtain an optimal recording.

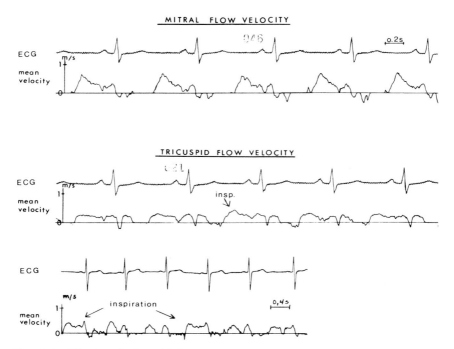

Fig. 4–4. Mitral and tricuspid flow velocity curves from normal subjects recorded with pulsed Doppler. Mitral flow velocity is higher in early diastole and has a more rapid decline. Tricuspid flow velocity is lower, with a slower decline and with respiratory variation. Systolic flow velocity in the right ventricle is positive when transducer direction is toward the tricuspid valve area.

This difference in flow velocity patterns through the two atrioventricular valves is also easily seen in children and infants. In newborns and in infants, in whom the heart rate is high and the diastole is short, the difference may be less obvious, but still clear enough as shown in Figure 4.5. Mitral flow velocity is highest in early diastole and decreases clearly before atrial contraction causes the second peak. Tricuspid flow velocity is lower in early

NORMAL INFANTS

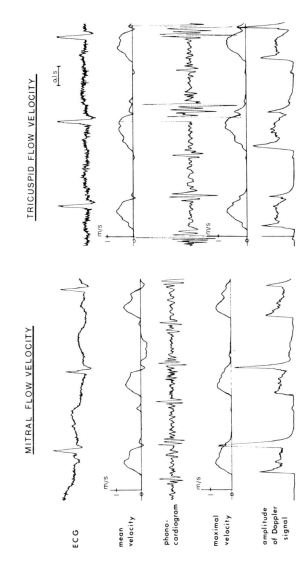

Fig. 4–5. Pulsed Doppler recording from infants 2 to 3 weeks old. Mitral flow velocity is highest in early diastole; tricuspid flow velocity is highest following atrial contraction. The earlier opening and later closure of the tricuspid valve are seen.

65

diastole, there is no decrease before atrial contraction, and the second peak is invariably the highest in this age group. This may be partly due to the short diastole, but may also be caused by the physiologic right ventricular hypertrophy present at birth, since similar velocity curves are recorded in children and adults with right ventricular hypertrophy.

When the transducer is directed toward the tricuspid orifice, recording in the right ventricle close to the valve shows flow velocity toward the transducer in both diastole and systole. When the beam is directed up toward the right ventricular outflow tract, velocity of flow in systole is away from the transducer as in the left ventricle.

When the best direction for recording velocity of flow into the right ventricle is found, the sample volume is moved gradually toward the tricuspid orifice. First, only blood flow is recorded. Next are recorded the tricuspid valve opening and at the orifice both valve opening and closure, in addition to the flow velocity (Figure 4.6). Further back into the right atrium forward diastolic flow velocity is less clearly recorded, but may be clearly heard during inspiration. With increased flow in the right atrium, velocity of flow toward the transducer in diastole can be recorded almost as well as into the right ventricle. In the presence of atrial septal defects with significant left-to-right shunting, velocity of flow toward the transducer can be recorded in both systole and diastole in the right atrium. Even in such cases, right atrial and right ventricular flow velocities can be easily separated by recording the valve movements in the direction through the valve orifice.

D. Pulmonary Valve Area

The velocity of flow in the right ventricle in systole can be followed up into the outflow tract and into the pulmonary artery. A position at the left sternal border in the fourth or fifth intercostal space or the subcostal position usually gives the highest velocity in the outflow tract. For optimal recording of flow velocity in the pulmonary artery, a position one or two intercostal spaces higher up may be better. When the sample volume is moved up toward the pulmonary artery, a similar pattern as in the left ventricle is found (Figure 4.7). At first, valve closure is recorded in addition to flow velocity. Then both valve opening and closure and a slight change in the flow velocity curve are recorded. Above this level, the sound of valve closure disappears first, then also the valve opening.

In the pulmonary artery, especially in children and young adults, flow away from the transducer may be recorded in late diastole during inspiration (Figure 4.8). This may represent diastolic flow into the pulmonary artery following atrial contraction. In subjects with low diastolic pressure, as in pulmonary regurgitation, this may also be seen during expiration, as shown in the lower part of Figure 4.8. When one is recording velocity only in the right ventricular outflow tract, this can be difficult or impossible to distin-

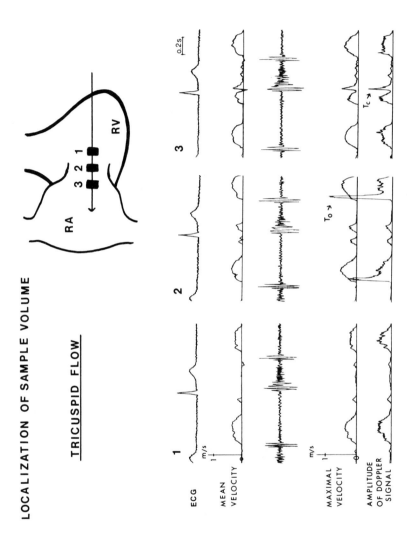

Fig. 4–6. Pulsed Doppler recording of tricuspid flow velocity. When the sample volume is moving toward the tricuspid orifice, tricuspid valve opening (To) is first recorded (2). At the orifice (3) only the valve closure (Tc) is recorded. In a position between 2 and 3, both opening and closure would be recorded. Increase in velocity with atrial contraction is better recorded close to the valve than further into the right ventricle. RA—right atrium; RV—right ventricle.

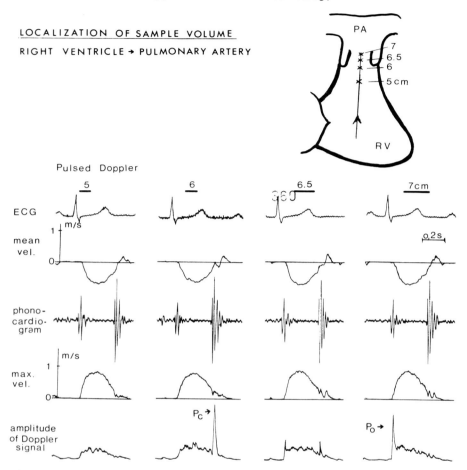

Fig. 4–7. Pulsed Doppler recording of flow velocity in the right ventricle and pulmonary valve area. With transducer direction toward the outflow tract, flow is away from the transducer in systole. At 5 cm valve movements are not recorded. At 6 cm pulmonary valve closure (P$_c$) is noted, at 6.5 cm both valve opening and closure are recorded, and higher up the valve opening (P$_o$) is best recorded. PA—pulmonary artery; RV—right ventricle.

guish from the velocity in the left ventricular outflow tract. These can be distinguished, however, by following the blood flow up into the arteries and 1) locating the pulmonary valve to the right and above the aortic valve (provided relations of the great vessels are normal), 2) timing the pulmonary valve closure compared to the second component of the second heart sound (provided conditions causing reverse splitting of the second heart sound are not present) and 3) observing the different velocity curve forms in the aorta

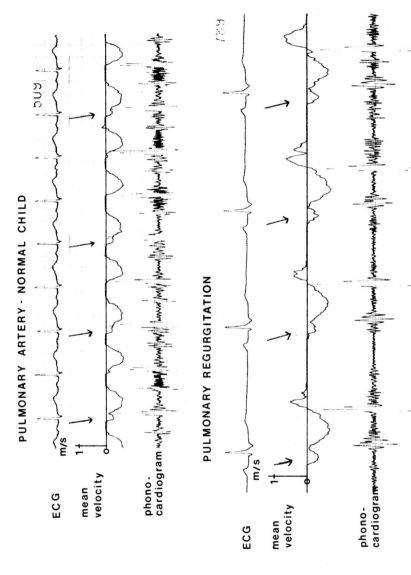

Fig. 4-8. During inspiration flow velocity away from the transducer is seen in late diastole (arrows), probably following right atrial contraction. With pulmonary regurgitation and a low pulmonary artery diastolic pressure, this pattern may be recorded also during expiration (lower curve). The positive velocity recorded in early diastole represents pulmonary regurgitation. Both curves are recorded with pulsed Doppler.

69

and the pulmonary artery. The velocity of flow can also be followed from the respective atrioventricular valves and to the great arteries as described.

E. Flow Velocity Recorded from the Suprasternal Notch

Figure 4.9 shows the difference in velocity curve forms of the ascending aorta and the pulmonary artery in a normal subject. Velocity is higher in the aorta and shows a more rapid increase, with peak velocity earlier in systole than in the pulmonary artery. The same difference in flow velocity signals and in curve form is found whether velocity in the two great arteries is recorded from the apex, the left sternal border, or the suprasternal notch. To record flow in the ascending aorta, one usually directs the transducer a little forward and to the right, and for the descending aorta, backward and a little to the left. The pulmonary artery can be reached by directing the transducer straight forward from the descending aorta or to the left from the ascending aorta as shown in Figure 4.10. The recording here is first from the pulmonary artery, and then by angling to the right from the ascending aorta and back to the pulmonary artery. The difference in velocity curves is also seen here, but

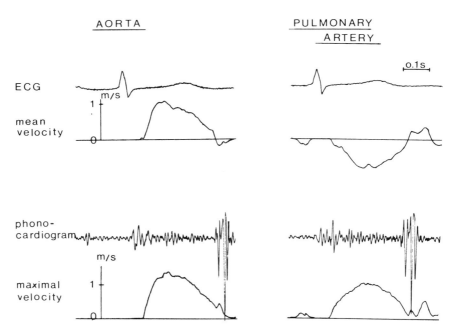

Fig. 4–9. Pulsed Doppler recording of flow velocity in the ascending aorta recorded from the suprasternal notch and in the pulmonary artery recorded from the left sternal border. Velocity in the aorta is higher and increase in velocity in early systole is more rapid. The flow velocity curve from the pulmonary artery is more rounded with a later peak velocity.

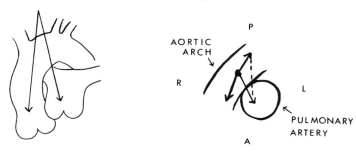

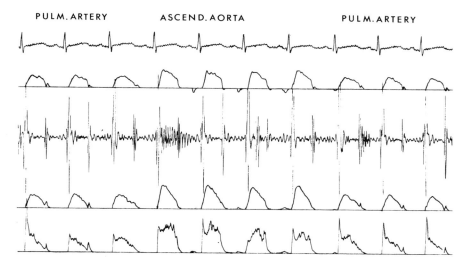

Fig. 4–10. Pulsed Doppler recording from the suprasternal notch shows a scan from the pulmonary artery to the aorta and back to the pulmonary artery. The latter is usually easiest to find by angling the transducer anteriorly from the descending aorta. To ascertain that a recorded flow velocity is from the pulmonary artery, one should move the sample volume down to the valve level to record pulmonary valve closure. In the two first and last beats, valve closure coincides with the second component of the second heart sound. For aortic valve closure to be recorded, the sample volume has to be moved a little lower in the aorta. A—anterior; P—posterior; L—left; R—right.

to ascertain the position in the respective arteries, the sample volume should be moved down toward the valve level to also record the valve closures. When one is recording from above and moving the sample volume down toward the valve level, the opening movement is recorded first, then both opening and closure, and further down into the respective ventricles only valve closures are recorded.

F. Maximal Velocities in Normal Subjects

Table 4.1 shows the average and the range of maximal velocities recorded in 30 normal children from 1 to 16 years of age and in 40 adults from 18 to 72 years of age. Higher velocities were usually found in children. Among the adults, velocities were lower in the older patients. Tricuspid flow velocity may be somewhat overestimated compared to mitral flow velocity since maximal velocity through the tricuspid valve was measured during inspiration and averaging over one or more respiratory cycles was not done.

4.4   COMMENTS

The velocity curves in the various parts of the heart are characteristic enough to allow recognition in normal individuals, but in pathologic conditions they may be sufficiently changed to make this difficult or impossible. The position of the various velocity patterns in relation to the chest wall is also characteristic in normal individuals, but in patients with congenital heart disease with abnormal chamber positions or relations this may not be of any help. Even in such cases, however, the tricuspid valve can usually be identified by noting the effect of respiration on velocity of flow through the valve. Since the velocity of flow into a ventricle can be followed up into the outflow part and into the respective artery, the flow from an atrioventricular valve and into an artery can be shown. Whether this artery is the aorta or the pulmonary artery may be shown by comparing measurements made from the apex with measurements from the suprasternal notch where flow in the ascending aorta can be recorded above the pulmonary artery and followed into the descending aorta. Use of the time relation between the aortic/pulmonary valve closure and the simultaneously recorded phonocardiogram may also be helpful. Therefore, in most cases localization of the sample volume can be achieved by use of Doppler without a simultaneous echocardiogram, and is easily accomplished in most subjects. Echocardiograms taken before or following the Doppler recording may be helpful, but

Table 4.1   Maximal Velocities Recorded Noninvasively With Doppler Ultrasound in Normal Individuals (m/s)

	Children	Adults
Mitral flow	1.00 (0.8–1.3)	0.90 (0.6–1.3)
Tricuspid flow	0.60 (0.5–0.8)	0.50 (0.3–0.7)
Pulmonary artery	0.90 (0.7–1.1)	0.75 (0.6–0.9)
Left ventricle	1.00 (0.7–1.2)	0.90 (0.7–1.1)
Aorta	1.50 (1.2–1.8)	1.35 (1.0–1.7)

in patients with complex anatomy, simultaneous use of the two methods may be necessary for unambiguous localization.

The advantage of using Doppler without the aid of simultaneous M-mode echo is that small angles or alignment between ultrasound beam and velocity direction are easier to obtain. To only detect the presence of abnormal flow, the angle between velocity and ultrasound beam is of less importance. With small angles giving optimal Doppler signals, however, velocity of blood flow can be obtained and the direction of velocity can be better established than as merely toward or away from the transducer.

Combining Doppler and two-dimensional echo can be of help since the latter, in addition to localization of the sample volume, may help to obtain a small angle to a velocity by indicating the direction of blood flow. Although this could be helpful with flow through normal and possibly also stenotic valves, the direction of a regurgitant jet might not be possible to infer. Therefore, for one to obtain optimal Doppler signals, the need for orienting the ultrasound beam from the quality of the Doppler signal would still be present.

A pulsed Doppler alone can be sufficient to record velocity of blood flow in the heart and great vessels in most normal subjects, even if orientation may be more convenient if combined with CW Doppler. In some young individuals, velocity of flow in the ascending aorta may exceed the limit of 1.75 m/s for the pulsed mode, and when one is recording velocities between 8 and 12 cm depth in adults, the limit of 1 m/s may sometimes be exceeded. In most pathologic conditions, however, velocities exceed the limit for the pulsed mode, and the CW mode is necessary to obtain these.

The described sequence of valve movements is found when recording in the direction of the blood flow; it is not necessarily found if recording at a transverse angle to the valve. The angle to the blood flow is also important when attempting to record velocity of the flow. It may not always be possible to obtain a small enough angle to the blood flow in the chambers or valve areas to record maximal velocity of the blood flow. However, even with angles up to 30°, underestimation of velocity is within 13%. For measurements in the aortic arch or descending aorta, comparison with roentgenograms has indicated that small angles can usually be obtained.[9] Good correlations have also been shown between velocities obtained noninvasively with Doppler and by electromagnetic flow meters both in experimental animals[9] and in man.[6]

The maximal velocities reported here are in the same range as those reported by others in the aorta[7,9] and in the pulmonary artery.[4] The lower velocities regularly recorded in the pulmonary artery compared to the aorta are consistent with the lower peak pressure drop present in early systole across the pulmonary valve. Using high-fidelity catheter-tip transducers, Murgo, et al. recorded at rest a peak pressure drop early in systole of 3.8 mm

Hg across the pulmonary valve and 7.5 mm Hg across the aortic valve, with increase during exercise to 6.5 and 12.4 mm Hg respectively.[14] In valvular obstructions, increases in maximal velocity across the obstruction have been used to calculate the pressure drop across the obstruction.[11,15] If the same method is used to calculate a peak pressure drop from increase in maximal velocity across normal aortic valves, values close to those reported by Murgo, et al. are obtained. (Increase in maximal velocity from 0.80 m/s in the left ventricle to 1.50 m/s in the aorta gives a calculated peak pressure drop of 6.5 mm Hg.) With exercise, increases in velocity comparable to the increases in peak pressure drop reported by Murgo, et al. can also be recorded.

The difference in the flow velocity curve forms in the aorta and the pulmonary artery has also been described through recording with electromagnetic flow meters in experimental animals[16] and in humans.[14] This is most likely due to the lower vascular resistance in the pulmonary circulation, since increases in pulmonary vascular resistance make the pulmonary flow velocity curve more like that in the aorta.[17] The difference in mitral and tricuspid flow velocity curves recorded in normal subjects may also be due to the difference in pressure drop across the valves. With left atrial pressure higher than right atrial, a slightly higher pressure difference may be present early in diastole between atrium and ventricle in the left heart and may cause the higher peak velocity of flow through the mitral valve.

REFERENCES

1. Johnson S.L., Baker D.W., Lute R.A., Dodge H.T.: Doppler echocardiography. The localization of cardiac murmurs. Circulation 1973; 48: 810-822.
2. Baker D.W., Rubenstein S.A., Lorch G.S.: Pulsed Doppler echocardiography—principles and applications. Am. J. Med. 1977; 63: 69-80.
3. Matsuo H., Kitabatake A., Hayashi T., Asao M., Terao Y., Senda S., Hamanaka Y., Matsumoto M., Nimura Y., Abe H.: Intracardiac flow dynamics with bidirectional ultrasonic pulsed Doppler. Jpn. Circ. J. 1977; 41: 515-528.
4. Griffith J.M., Henry W.L.: An ultrasound system for combined cardiac imaging and Doppler blood flow measurement in man. Circulation 1978; 57: 925-930.
5. Light L.H.: Transcutaneous aortovelography—a new window on the circulation? Br. Heart J. 1976; 38: 433-442.
6. Sequeira R.F., Light L.H., Cross G., Raftery E.B.: Transcutaneous aortovelography: A quantitative evaluation. Br. Heart J. 1976; 38: 443-450.
7. Fraser C.B., Light L.H., Shinebourne E.A., Buchthal A., Healy M.J.R., Beardshaw J.A.: Transcutaneous aortovelography: reproducibility in adults and children. Eur. J. Cardiol. 1976; 4: 181-189.
8. Boughner D.R.: Assessment of aortic insufficiency by transcutaneous Doppler ultrasound. Circulation 1975; 52: 874-879.
9. Huntsman L.L., Gams E., Johnson C.C., Fairbanks E.: Transcutaneous determination of aortic blood-flow velocities in man. Am. Heart J. 1975; 89: 605-612.
10. Angelsen B.A.J., Brubakk A.O.: Transcutaneous measurement of blood flow velocity in the human aorta. Cardiovasc. Res. 1976; 10: 368-379.
11. Holen J., Aaslid R., Landmark K., Simonsen S.: Determination of pressure gradient in mitral stenosis with a non-invasive ultrasound Doppler technique. Acta Med. Scand. 1976; 199: 455-460.

12. Brubakk A.O., Angelsen B.A.J., Hatle L.: Diagnosis of valvular heart disease using transcutaneous Doppler ultrasound. Cardiovasc. Res. 1977; 11: 461-469.
13. Yoshida T., Mori M., Nimura Y., Hikita G., Takagishi S., Nakanishi K., Satomura S.: Analysis of heart motion with ultrasonic Doppler method and its clinical application. Am. Heart J. 1961; 61: 61-75.
14. Murgo J.P., Altobelli S.A., Dorethy J.F., Logsdon J.R., McGranahan G.H.: Normal ventricular ejection dynamics in man during rest and exercise. *In*: Physiologic Principles of Heart Sounds and Murmurs. Edited by Leon S.F., Shaver J.A. Dallas, American Heart Association 1975; 92-101.
15. Hatle L., Brubakk A., Tromsdal A., Angelsen B.: Noninvasive assessment of pressure drop in mitral stenosis by Doppler ultrasound. Br. Heart J. 1978; 40: 131-140.
16. Franklin D.L., van Citters R.L., Rushmer R.F.: Balance between right and left ventricular output. Circ. Res. 1962; 10: 17-26.
17. Hatle L.: Changes in pulmonary flow velocity curves in pulmonary hypertension. To be published.

5

Pulsed and Continuous Wave Doppler in Diagnosis and Assessment of Various Heart Lesions

5.1 INTRODUCTION

To obtain the velocity of blood flow within the heart noninvasively with Doppler ultrasound, alignment or a small angle ($<30°$) between the ultrasound beam and velocity direction is necessary (see Section 4.2). The area of pulsed Doppler recording can be localized from valve movements and the velocity patterns obtained as described in the previous chapter. By moving the sample volume in the direction of the blood flow in the valve areas, one can diagnose obstructions to blood flow from localized increases in velocity and valve regurgitations from reversal of blood flow at the valve areas and into the chamber behind.

To obtain increased velocities it is necessary to use continuous wave (CW) Doppler as discussed in Sections 3.3 and 3.6. Obstructions can be quantitated from the maximal velocities obtained together with the time course of the velocity curve.[1-6] Increases in velocity can also be found in the absence of obstructions, when the flow is increased. In this chapter we describe the diagnosis of regurgitations; the diagnosis, localization, and assessment of obstructions; and the differentiation between increased velocity caused by obstructions or by increased flow. Some other changes in velocity curves and the Doppler signals from valve motions are described.

Pulsed Doppler was used to localize Doppler signals and to record velocities within the limit for this mode. CW Doppler was used for orientation and to detect and record high velocities. For all the velocity patterns, attempts were made to record with the smallest angle to the velocity that could be found.

The experience described derives from Doppler recording in normal subjects as well as in a large number of patients with various heart diseases.

76

5.2 OBSTRUCTIONS TO FLOW

When obstructions to blood flow are present, velocity of flow increases. The increase in velocity requires a pressure drop across the obstruction. The approximate pressure drop can be calculated using Equation 2.2: $p_1 - p_2 = 4 \cdot v^2$ where $p_1 - p_2$ is the pressure drop and v is maximal velocity across the obstruction.

If the velocity proximal to an obstruction is also high, then this has to be considered in calculating the pressure drop, using Equation 2.24.

Viscous losses as well as inertia may also have to be considered. This is discussed in Section 2.4A. If viscous losses cannot be neglected, the pressure drop calculated from the maximal velocities will be too low. With in vitro experiments, Holen[7] has shown the relation between pressure drop and velocity to be valid for orifices of a diameter of 8 mm (area 0.5 cm²). With diameters of 1.5 and 3.5 mm (areas $\leq$ 0.1 cm²), velocity measurements underestimated the pressure drop. The greatest underestimation was seen with the smallest orifice and with low pressure drops. This might be due to viscous losses becoming more important with smaller orifices. For the valve areas usually seen in valvular obstructions, decreases in velocity due to viscous losses are probably not important.

During rapid increases in velocity, a delay in velocity compared to the pressure drop due to inertia might be expected. Murgo, et al. have shown that an increase in velocity is delayed compared to the simultaneously recorded pressure drop across normal aortic and pulmonary valves.[8] A similar delay between pressure drop and velocity has been recorded in aortic valve stenosis.[5] This may be significant if calculation of a mean pressure drop from the maximal velocity curve is attempted. The magnitude of the peak pressure drop is not significantly influenced by this delay. This is discussed in more detail in Section 2.4A.

To record the increased velocity across an obstruction noninvasively with Doppler, alignment or a small angle to the velocity is necessary; otherwise, velocity and pressure drop will be underestimated. Figure 5.1 illustrates the degree of underestimation that occurs with increasing angles between ultrasound beam and velocity. Since the pressure drop is obtained by squaring the velocity, underestimation of pressure drop is larger. A velocity of 2 m/s gives a pressure drop of 16 mm Hg. An angle of 10° gives 15.5 mm Hg (97%), a 30° angle gives 12 mm Hg (75%), and with 60° a pressure drop of 4 mm Hg (25%) is obtained.

A. Mitral Stenosis

In mitral stenosis the pressure drop calculated from the noninvasive recording of maximal velocity in the mitral jet correlates well with pressures recorded at catheterization.[1-4] This experience indicates that a small angle to the mitral jet can be obtained quite easily in almost all patients with mitral stenosis.

EFFECT OF ANGLE TO VELOCITY

ON RECORDED VELOCITY

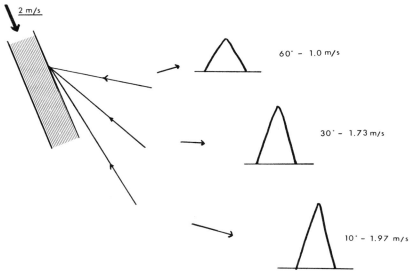

Fig. 5–1. With an angle of 60° between ultrasound beam and velocity, the velocity estimated from the frequency shift alone is only half the velocity present. At 10° the underestimation of velocity is negligible.

Velocity of mitral flow is usually best recorded from the apical area with the transducer directed toward the back and slightly upward. With mitral stenosis and increased velocity across the valve, higher frequencies are present in the audio signal which makes it clearly different from the audio signal of normal mitral flow velocity. When the Doppler signal of mitral flow velocity is obtained, the transducer is moved and angled while one is listening to the audio signal until the position with the highest frequencies is found. This represents the direction with the smallest angle to the jet.

Figure 5.2 shows mitral flow velocity in a normal subject on the left. Maximum velocity is close to 1 m/s in early diastole and decreases rapidly. In the patient with mitral stenosis, maximum velocity is above 2 m/s. It decreases slowly and, with the increase following atrial contraction, is still greater than 1 m/s at the end of diastole. The calculated pressure drop during diastole is shown at the bottom for each beat. With exercise (bicycling in the supine position), increase in velocity occurs almost instantaneously. With increased heart rate, atrial contraction may occur so early in diastole that the second peak may no longer be clearly distinguished and the decline in velocity early in diastole is no longer seen. Doppler signals from the mitral

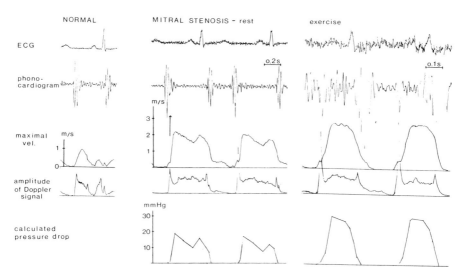

Fig. 5–2. Maximal velocity of mitral flow recorded with pulsed Doppler in a normal subject and with CW Doppler in a patient with mitral stenosis at rest and during exercise. In mitral stenosis maximal velocity is higher, decline in velocity is slower, and a significant pressure drop is present throughout diastole. The amplitude curve shows the early opening of the mitral valve with the opening snap in the phonocardiogram not clearly separated from the second heart sound. With exercise, heart rate increases from 70 to 126 and a clear increase in maximal velocity and calculated pressure drop is found.

jet are easily obtained also during exercise, but with increased respiration good signals may only be recorded intermittently.

In Figure 5.3 the pressure drop calculated from the maximal velocity recorded is compared to the pressure drop obtained at catheterization. With a good Doppler signal the two compare well. With an inferior signal (i.e., with more lower frequencies) as in the fifth beat, maximal velocity and pressure drop are underestimated. The increase in maximal velocity and calculated pressure drop with atrial contraction is not shown in the pressure recording, possibly because the pulmonary capillary wedge pressure does not show an increase in left atrial pressure with atrial contraction in this patient. With transseptal catheterization and recording of left atrial and left ventricular pressures, the increase in pressure drop with atrial contraction was clearly seen also from the pressure recording.[4]

Figure 5.4 shows the close correlation between mean diastolic pressure drop calculated from maximal velocity recorded during cardiac catheterization and the pressure drop obtained by pressure recording in 33 patients. Some of these data have been published earlier.[1,2] Repeated measurements

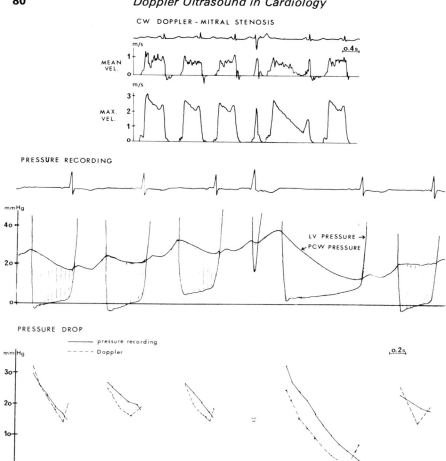

Fig. 5–3.   Maximal velocity recorded from the mitral jet with CW Doppler together with left ventricular (LV) and pulmonary capillary wedge (PCW) pressure in a patient with mitral stenosis. The pressure drops obtained by the two methods are compared. In the fifth beat, mean velocity is more poorly recorded suggesting that less of the mitral jet is traversed by the ultrasound beam, and for this beat calculated pressure drop is lower than that recorded by pressure. Note that effect of atrial contraction is clearly seen in the maximal velocity curve, but does not show clearly in the pressure curve.

with Doppler may show quite large day-to-day variations in pressure drop, especially in atrial fibrillation where heart rate may show greater variations. When a pressure drop is obtained at a certain heart rate at one examination, a higher or lower pressure drop at a subsequent examination is usually associated with a higher or a lower heart rate. In the follow-up of patients, the heart rate at the examination is essential in comparing pressure drops if changes in severity of the obstruction are to be assessed.

In contrast to Figure 5.4, Figure 5.5 shows the differences in pressure drop between Doppler and catheterization data in 18 patients for whom measurements were taken on different days. When the two methods differed significantly, heart rate was also clearly different on the two occasions.

A low or high pressure drop across the valve may be found whether the obstruction is mild or severe, depending upon the flow across the valve. The slope of the maximum velocity curve is influenced by the degree of obstruction, with a mild obstruction pressure drop and maximal velocity decreases occurring more rapidly than when obstruction is severe. The time-course of

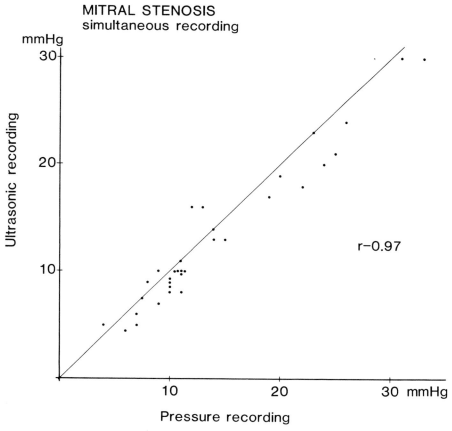

Fig. 5–4. **Mean diastolic pressure drop calculated from maximal velocity of mitral flow compared to pressure drop recorded simultaneously at catheterization in 33 patients with mitral stenosis or combined mitral stenosis and regurgitation.**

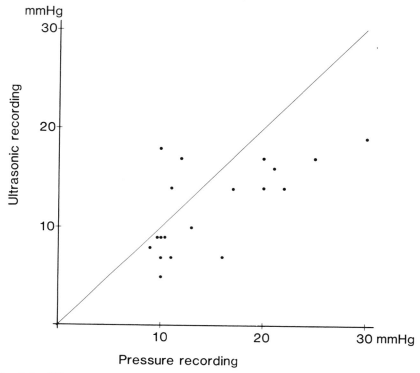

MITRAL STENOSIS
nonsimultaneous recording

Fig. 5–5. When measurements are taken on separate days, greater differences between the two methods are found, but with differences in pressure drop, heart rate on the two occasions varies similarly.

the pressure difference can be expressed as the pressure half-time, i.e., the time it takes until the initial pressure drop is halved. Since the relationship between velocity and pressure drop is quadratic, pressure half-time can be obtained directly from the maximal velocity curve by dividing peak velocity by 1.4 ($\sim\sqrt{2}$) and measuring the time from peak velocity to where this decrease in velocity is found. Pressure half-time was found to correlate with mitral valve area and to be relatively independent of flow across the valve.[2] Pressure half-times were < 60 ms in normal individuals and 100 to 400 ms in subjects with mitral stenosis, increasing with decreasing valve area. With a pressure half-time > 220 ms, a valve area < 1.0 cm² was found.

From these data the following formula was used to estimate mitral valve area (MVA) from the noninvasively recorded pressure half-time in 20 additional patients with mitral stenosis:

$$\text{MVA (cm}^2) = \frac{220}{\textbf{pressure half-time (ms)}}$$

The results are shown in Figure 5.6. The correlation between mitral valve area estimated from the maximal velocity curve and the valve area calculated from catheterization data was 0.87. A good estimate of mitral valve area from the maximal mitral flow velocity curve, therefore, seems possible. The method should be equally useful in patients with associated mitral regurgitation where presence of a high pressure drop may be mainly due to either large flow across the valve or pronounced obstruction. A short or long pressure half-time may then indicate whether regurgitation or obstruction is the main lesion. It is also useful to indicate the severity of obstruction in patients with severe mitral stenosis and low cardiac output where a low pressure drop might lead to underestimation of the degree of obstruction.

With exercise (bicycling in the supine position), a moderate decrease in pressure half-time is usually seen. Figure 5.7 shows the effect of exercise on

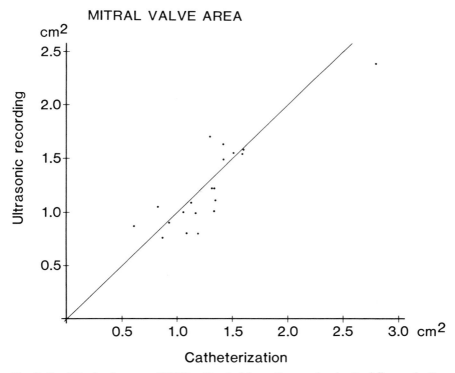

Fig. 5–6. Mitral valve area (MVA) estimated from the maximal mitral flow velocity curve and compared to MVA calculated from catheterization data in 20 patients with mitral stenosis.

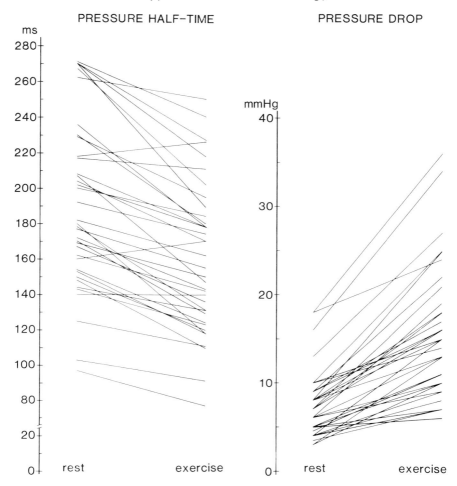

Fig. 5–7. Changes in pressure half-time and mean diastolic pressure drop with exercise in 37 patients with mitral stenosis or combined stenosis and regurgitation. There is a moderate decrease in pressure half-time with exercise (from 190 to 160 ms, P < 0.001) while the simultaneous increase in pressure drop is more pronounced (from 7.6 to 16 mm Hg).

pressure half-time and mean diastolic pressure drop in 37 patients. Pressure half-time decreases from a mean of 190 ms to 160 ms (P < 0.001). This indicates that increase in flow may lead to a decrease in pressure half-time, but the change in pressure half-time is moderate compared to the much greater change in pressure drop with exercise. An experimental study has also shown decrease in pressure half-time with increase in flow.[9]

Figure 5.8 shows the decline in maximal velocity during diastole in three different patients with mitral stenosis. The slope of the maximal velocity

MITRAL STENOSIS

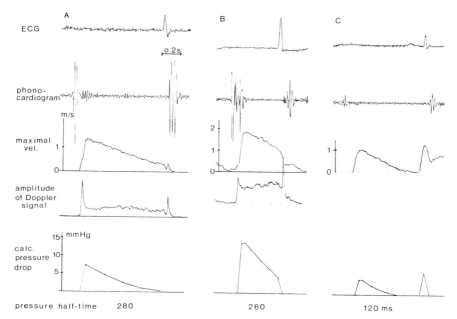

Fig. 5–8. Patients A and B have tight mitral stenosis (MVA < 1 cm²) and atrial fibrillation. Patient C has mild mitral stenosis and sinus bradycardia. Pressure half-time is very long in patient A and B, and only slightly prolonged in patient C. Note that the slope of the velocity curve is similar in B and C, but the pressure half-time is much longer in B owing to the higher velocity. Maximal velocity in A is only slightly higher than in C, but the longer pressure half-time indicates that the severity of obstruction is greater than in C.

curve may resemble the slope of the anterior mitral valve recorded with M-mode echocardiography. Calculation of the pressure half-time, however, shows that similar slopes give widely different pressure half-times depending upon the height of the maximal velocity curve in early diastole. The higher the maximal velocity, the steeper the slope may be, and pressure half-time may still be significantly prolonged. When maximal velocity is low, pressure half-time can be only slightly prolonged; consequently, obstruction is mild despite a nearly horizontal slope of the velocity curve (Figure 5.8C). Pressure half-times are similar in A and B. The difference in pressure drop is due to low cardiac output in A. It is normal in B.

Since the maximal velocity curve gives the pressure drop across the valve and the rate of decrease of pressure drop during diastole indicates the degree of obstruction, calculation of both indicates flow across the valve. Increase in velocity across the mitral valve can also be found in the absence of mitral valve disease when flow across the valve is greatly increased. Figure 5.9 is

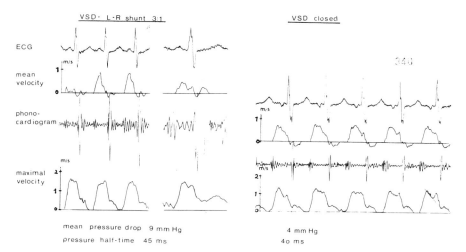

Fig. 5–9. **Increased velocity of flow across the mitral valve in a child with ventricular septal defect and a left to right shunt of 3:1. Pressure half-time is in the normal range. Following operation, velocity decreased, but was still higher than expected. A residual shunt was later shown to be present. A similar pressure drop was found at catheterization and at operation the mitral valve was normal.**

from a child with a ventricular septal defect and a left-to-right shunt of 3:1. Maximal velocity of mitral flow gave a calculated mean pressure drop across the valve of 9 mm Hg. A similar pressure drop was found at catheterization. Pressure half-time calculated from the velocity curve was 45 ms, which is normal, indicating that there was no obstruction and that the high velocity and increased pressure drop were due to increased flow. At operation there was no obstruction at the mitral valve area, and following closure of the ventricular septal defect, lower velocities across the mitral valve were recorded.

In mild mitral stenosis or mitral stenosis with low cardiac output, maximal velocity of flow across the valve may be within the limits for the pulsed mode. When more than mild obstruction is present, however, maximal velocity exceeds the limit for the pulsed mode. Figure 5.10 shows how the maximal velocity in such cases is lost when the pulsed mode is used. It also shows the artifacts that occur in the mean velocity curve (negative deflection despite direction of flow toward the transducer) when velocities above the limit for the pulsed mode are present (see Figure 3.19, Section 3.6). Assessments of the degree of mitral stenosis with pulsed Doppler have been described, using these artifacts and their duration during diastole as an indication of the severity of mitral stenosis.[10, 11] The artifacts only indicate that

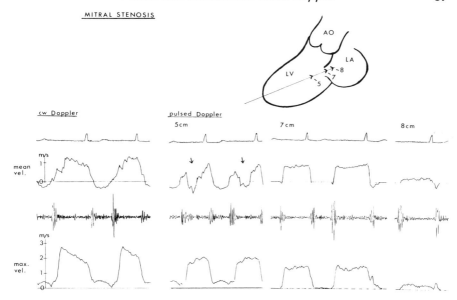

Fig. 5–10.   CW and pulsed Doppler recording of mean and maximal velocity of mitral flow in a patient with mitral stenosis. The CW mode shows that maximal velocity is 2.8 m/s. With the pulsed mode velocities above 2 m/s are not recorded and the mean velocity curve shows artifacts (arrows) due to the presence of higher velocities than can be recorded with the pulsed mode. At 7 cm depth, toward the left atrium, maximal velocity is lower and the artifacts are no longer present. In the left atrium (8 cm) velocity is low. Mean velocity is directional and maximal velocity is nondirectional.

velocity at that time is above the limit for the method. Without the CW mode, the higher frequencies in the mitral jet are not heard, and the audio signal is then of less help in obtaining an optimal angle to the jet.

The good correlation reported between pressure drop calculated from maximal velocity recorded with CW Doppler and pressure drop recorded at catheterization[1-4] indicates that a small enough angle to the jet can usually be found in mitral stenosis. The audio signal is the guide to obtaining a small angle to a jet with high velocities. With alignment between the ultrasound beam and the velocity, the audio signal consists of almost entirely high frequencies. With increasing angles to the jet, more of the lower frequencies from lower velocities beside the jet are also present in the audio signal. This is illustrated in Figure 5.11. The difference between a small and a larger angle to the jet in the audio signal is easily heard. In the recorded curves the change from A to B is seen as a slight reduction in maximal velocity and a relatively greater reduction in mean velocity because more of the lower frequencies are present in the signal. This difference is more easily seen if all the frequencies in the audio signal are recorded with spectral analysis, as shown in Figure 5.12.

Patients with left atrial myxomas obstructing the mitral orifice have a flow velocity pattern almost indistinguishable from that of mitral stenosis. In three patients with myxomas, mean diastolic pressure drops of 6, 14, and 20 mm Hg were calculated from the maximal velocities recorded. In addition to the Doppler signal from the increased velocity of flow, a lower frequent sound was heard at the beginning and at the end of diastole. It was simultaneous with, but of longer duration than, the valve opening and closure, and the sound differed clearly from the short, sharp clicks from the valve movements. With pulsed Doppler it was recorded in the left ventricle at the beginning of diastole and in the left atrium at the beginning of systole. This movement could be recorded clearly further back in the left atrium than the mitral valve closure. In two of the patients this finding strongly suggested the diagnosis of myxoma before an echocardiogram was taken. The patient with the highest pressure drop had pronounced flutter of the mitral valve throughout diastole. At echocardiography and at operation the mitral valve in this patient seemed stretched around a myxoma which almost completely occluded the mitral orifice in diastole.

The movement of left atrial myxomas has also been recorded by others using CW Doppler.[11a] In another report the recording of mitral flow with pulsed Doppler was considered normal in the mitral orifice while signs of disturbed flow were recorded in the left ventricle.[11b] The probable reason for this is that the first recording was on the atrial side of the orifice before the

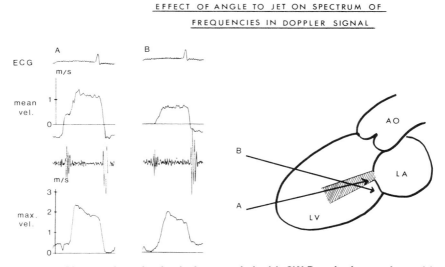

Fig. 5–11.   Mean and maximal velocity recorded with CW Doppler in a patient with mitral stenosis. A, A good audio signal indicates a small angle to the jet. In B high frequencies from the jet are still heard, but in addition the audio signal contains more low frequencies from beside the jet. Mean velocity is therefore lower.

MITRAL FLOW VELOCITY - MITRAL STENOSIS

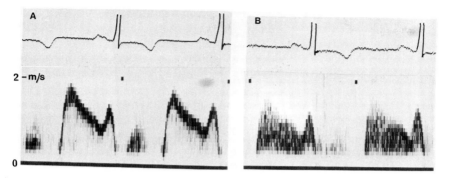

Fig. 5–12. **Spectral analysis of the Doppler signal from the mitral jet in a patient with mitral stenosis. A, A signal with mainly high frequencies (a clear tone-like signal). B, A more mixed signal with both high and low frequencies. Maximal velocity in B is only slightly lower than in A, but mean velocity would be much lower in B.**

occurrence of the clear increase in maximal velocity which would be present with a reported mean pressure drop of 16 mm Hg across the valve. Since only pulsed Doppler was used, only the disturbed flow was recorded in the left ventricle and not the increased velocity. Diastolic flutter of the mitral valve in left atrial myxoma has also been recorded with M-mode echocardiography.[11c]

B. Aortic Valve Stenosis

With CW Doppler it is also possible to record high velocities present in the aortic jet in aortic valve stenosis. The position where the highest velocities can be recorded varies. In children and young adults, best results are usually obtained from the suprasternal notch or the first right intercostal space. In older patients, the first or second right intercostal space is usually the best position. If the patient is turned over to the right side, Doppler signals from the ascending aorta can be obtained from the right sternal border in most patients with aortic valve stenosis. Occasionally, jet velocities are best recorded from the apex, left sternal border, third right intercostal space, or subcostal position.

Figure 5.13 compares aortic jet velocities in aortic stenosis to the velocity curve recorded in the ascending aorta in a normal subject. As in mitral stenosis, a peak pressure drop can be calculated from the maximal velocity recorded. The calculated peak pressure drop has been shown to correlate well with the peak pressure drop recorded at catheterization in young patients with aortic valve stenosis and somewhat less well in older patients where a good Doppler signal and a small angle to the aortic jet are not always obtained.[5, 6] Simultaneous measurements may show nearly identical

AORTIC FLOW VELOCITY

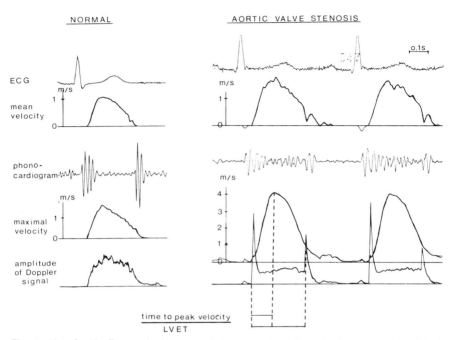

NORMAL   AORTIC VALVE STENOSIS

Fig. 5–13. Aortic flow velocity recorded with pulsed Doppler in a normal subject compared to velocity in aortic valve stenosis recorded with CW Doppler. In aortic stenosis maximal velocity recorded was 4.15 m/s and calculated peak pressure drop 68 mm Hg. Calculating the pressure drop for several points during systole gives a mean pressure drop of 38 mm Hg. In aortic valve stenosis, valve opening and closure are also recorded (CW Doppler) and show in the amplitude curve. In the normal subject, recording is from an area above the valve (pulsed Doppler) and valve movements not present in the Doppler signal. Peak of velocity in systole is later in aortic stenosis. Measurement of the time to peak velocity related to left ventricular ejection time (LVET) is shown.

peak pressure drops with the two methods, but the velocity curve is delayed compared to the pressure difference by pressure recording (Figure 5.14). A similar delay has been described between pressure drop and velocity of blood flow across normal aortic valves. Using high-fidelity catheter-tip transducers and an electromagnetic flow meter, Murgo, et al. recorded an interval of about 60 ms at rest in normal subjects between peak pressure drop and peak velocity in systole and a slightly shorter interval during exercise.[8] The delay in the flow velocity curve was ascribed to inertia.

The delay between the pressure recording and velocity recorded with Doppler in patients with aortic valve stenosis has been in the same range. Because of this delay, calculation of mean pressure drop during systole from

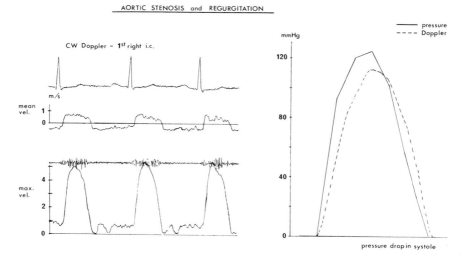

AORTIC STENOSIS and REGURGITATION

Fig. 5–14. **Comparison of the pressure drop across the aortic valve calculated from the recorded maximal velocity curve and recorded at catheterization in a patient with aortic stenosis and regurgitation. The delay in the velocity compared to the pressure recording is seen. The aortic regurgitation can be seen in the mean velocity curve as reverse flow in diastole, but the pulsed mode should be used for unambiguous recording of regurgitation.**

the maximal velocity curve may lead to an underestimation of the mean pressure drop even if maximal velocity in the jet has been recorded. It is not yet clear whether this delay may vary with the degree of obstruction across the valve or if it is constant enough to allow calculation of a mean pressure drop from the velocity curve.

As described with mitral stenosis, the audio signal is the guide to finding the best position and direction for recording from the aortic jet. Next to the jet, a harsh sound of high intensity is heard. If the ultrasound beam is directed toward the jet, higher frequencies are also present in the audio signal. With a direction where the ultrasound beam traverses the jet for some length (i.e., a small angle to the jet), the higher frequencies dominate the audio signal. A position may be obtained where mostly high frequencies are present in the audio signal and, with the high velocities that may be present in aortic valve stenosis, a clear high-frequency whistling sound may then be heard. It may have so high a frequency that it becomes almost inaudible. Thus, the quality of the audio signal may indicate whether a small angle to the jet has been obtained or not. In Figure 5.15 spectral analysis of the Doppler signal from the aortic jet in aortic valve stenosis shows how the distribution of velocities during systole may change when the beam direction is varied. In A, where a clear high-frequency sound was present, the greatest blackening is at the highest velocities, whereas in B lower frequencies dominate.

AORTIC STENOSIS - jet velocities

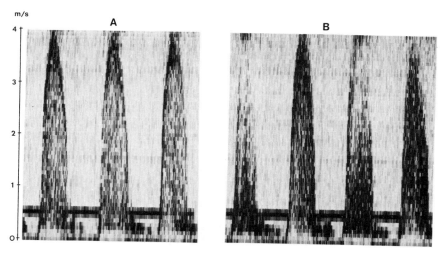

Fig. 5–15. Spectral analysis of Doppler signal from the aortic jet in aortic valve stenosis. A, A good Doppler signal with mainly high frequencies present. In the recording this shows as a strong blackening at the highest frequencies and at the edges during increase and decrease in velocity. B, A poorer Doppler signal. In the second beat, frequencies as high as in A are present, but also more of lower frequencies throughout systole. In the fourth beat there are still more of the lower frequencies and in the first and third beats the higher frequencies are partly lost.

The pressure drop calculated from the maximal velocity curve represents the peak pressure drop during systole. This may differ more or less from the pressure drop often reported from catheterization studies and measured as the difference between peak left ventricular and peak aortic pressures. These occur at different times during systole and should rather be called peak-to-peak pressure drop. As illustrated in Figure 5.16, the peak pressure drop is higher than that obtained by measuring from peak to peak. The difference between the two is largest in patients with mild to moderate aortic stenosis where the aortic pressure increases more during systole and the pressure difference decreases more towards end-systole. The difference is less in patients with more severe obstruction where the pressure difference is more maintained throughout systole.

The time in systole where the peak pressure difference occurs is seen to be later with increasing obstruction but, as shown in the last pressure tracing in Figure 5.16, the course of the left ventricular pressure curve also influences this measurement. With a more sustained left ventricular systolic pressure in this patient, peak pressure drop would have been later in systole. Therefore, in addition to differences in the severity of obstruction, changes in the left ventricular and aortic pressure curves from changes in contractility and

AORTIC STENOSIS   LV – AO PRESSURE DROP

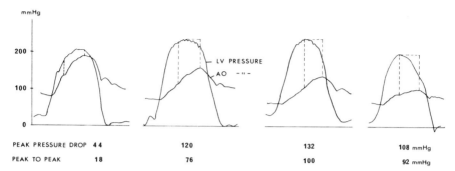

| PEAK PRESSURE DROP | 4 4 | 120 | 132 | 108 mmHg |
| PEAK TO PEAK | 18 | 76 | 100 | 92 mmHg |

Fig. 5–16. The difference between peak pressure drop as obtained from velocity recordings and the "peak-to-peak" pressure drop as often measured at catheterization is shown in four patients with aortic stenosis. The peak pressure drop is clearly higher and it occurs earlier in systole when obstruction is mild. With more severe obstruction the peak pressure drop comes later, and the difference between the two becomes less pronounced as the pressure drop is more maintained throughout systole.

peripheral resistance may influence the pressure difference and thus the course of the maximal velocity curve.

Figure 5.17 illustrates how the shape of the maximal velocity curve adds to the information of the peak pressure drop with a later peak velocity when the pressure difference is more sustained throughout systole. The time to

AORTIC VALVE STENOSIS

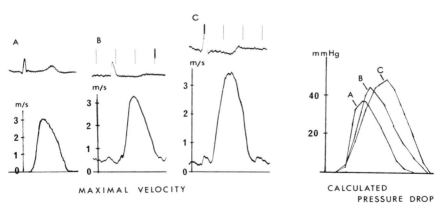

MAXIMAL VELOCITY   CALCULATED
                                      PRESSURE DROP

Fig. 5–17. Maximal velocity and calculated peak pressure drop differ only slightly in these three patients with aortic valve stenosis. In A there is an early peak and nearly equalization of pressures in late systole indicating insignificant obstruction. In B and C peak velocity occurs later in systole indicating more pronounced obstruction. A calculated mean pressure drop would also be considerably higher in C than in A.

peak velocity in systole is easiest to measure when aortic valve opening and closure are recorded together with the maximal velocity and with a paper speed of 100 mm/s as shown in Figure 5.13. The time to peak velocity can be expressed as a ratio of the left ventricular ejection time. With mild obstruction, this ratio is usually < 0.50, and with a ratio of 0.55 or more, obstruction is usually of a severity to indicate operation.[11d]

Measurement of the time of peak velocity in systole helps to avoid underestimation of the severity of obstruction in patients in whom a good Doppler signal cannot be found and in whom maximal velocity and pressure drop are underestimated.[5] Timing of peak velocity is often possible even if the velocity recorded is not very high. Care should be taken, however, that the Doppler signal is equally well recorded throughout systole, as shown in Figure 5.18.

In aortic valve stenosis velocities up to 6 m/s have been recorded with a calculated peak pressure drop of 144 mm Hg. Even in mild aortic stenosis, velocities exceed the limit for the pulsed mode. Assessments of aortic stenosis with pulsed Doppler have been described.[12-14] Some of the criteria used

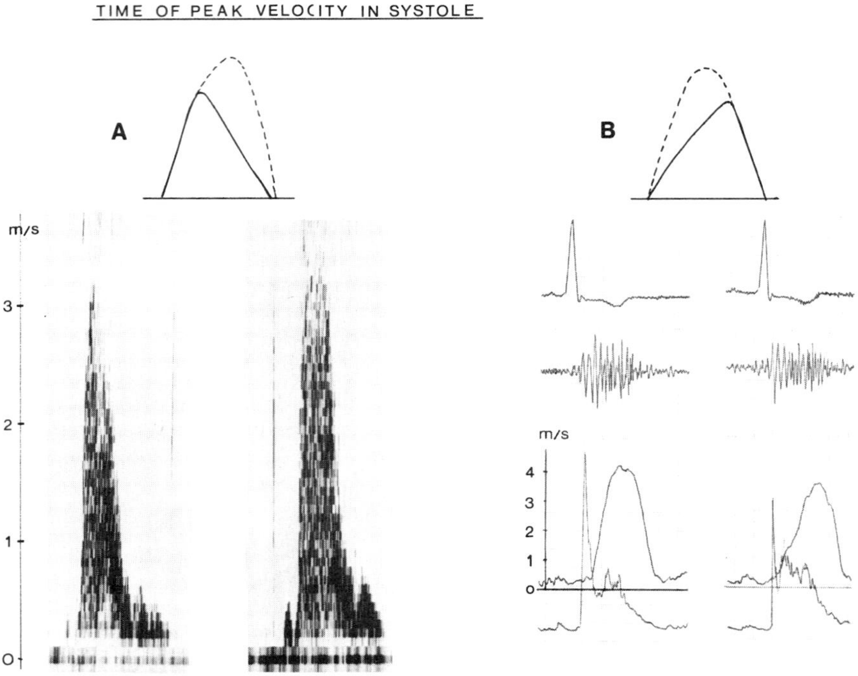

TIME OF PEAK VELOCITY IN SYSTOLE

Fig. 5–18. With a less than optimal Doppler signal from the jet, time of peak velocity in systole should only be measured if a rounded curve is clearly recorded throughout systole. With loss of part of the Doppler signal during systole a too early peak velocity would be obtained in the first beat in A and a too late peak velocity in the second beat in B. In the latter velocity is not clearly recorded in the first part of systole because of a fluttering aortic valve.

in this assessment, such as duration of negative velocities during systole and several peaks in the analogue signal, are artifacts introduced when velocities above the limit for the pulsed mode are present (see Section 3.6). Figure 5.19 shows an example of pulsed Doppler recording from the aortic jet in aortic stenosis. The repeated positive/negative shifts seen in the pulsed Doppler curve may indicate the presence of higher velocities during most of the systole, but these are only recorded if the sample volume is in the jet and with a reasonable angle to the velocity. The pulsed mode here was recorded after locating the jet with CW Doppler.

AORTIC VALVE STENOSIS

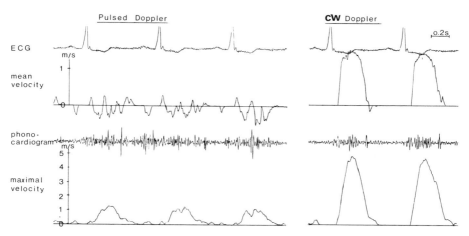

Fig. 5–19. Recording from aortic jet in aortic valve stenosis with pulsed and CW Doppler (same position and direction). Maximal velocity in the aortic jet is close to 5 m/s (calculated peak pressure drop 100 mm Hg). In the pulsed mode, velocities above 1 m/s cannot be recorded and the mean velocity curve shows several positive/negative shifts produced by the presence of higher velocities for the greater part of systole.

Pulsed Doppler can, however, be useful in the diagnosis or exclusion of aortic valve stenosis in patients with systolic murmurs.[14a,b] In many normal children and young adults, flow velocities in the aorta are above the limits for most pulsed Doppler systems producing artifacts in normal velocity curves, and this may cause some of the flow disturbances recorded in the aorta with pulsed Doppler in patients without aortic stenosis.[14c]

In aortic valve stenosis velocities recorded in the left ventricle in systole are usually within the normal range, and an increase in velocity is found at valve level or in patients with mobile, doming valves slightly higher as shown in Figure 5.20. In a few patients, moderately increased velocities can be recorded within the left ventricle. These are patients with hypertrophic,

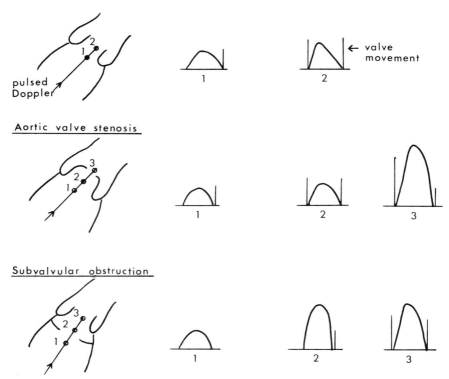

Fig. 5–20.   The change in the flow velocity patterns below and at the aortic valve area with valvular and subvalvular obstruction. In normal individuals a slight increase in velocity and change in the flow velocity curve are recorded at a level where both valve opening and closure are equally well recorded. In valvular stenosis increase in velocity is detected at the same level when valve movement is restricted, and higher up where valve opening is best recorded with a mobile doming valve. In subvalvular obstruction, increase in velocity is found at a level where only valve closure or no valve movements are recorded.

nondilated left ventricles where a moderate intraventricular pressure drop may develop secondary to the hypertrophy. The velocity curve in the left ventricle in these patients is characteristic with a late systolic maximum instead of the normal rounded curve (see Figure 5.51). There may be an abrupt decrease in velocity before end-systole in the lower part of the left ventricle corresponding to the near emptying or cavity obliteration that can be seen on angiocardiograms or with two-dimensional echo. Similar changes are seen in patients with hypertrophic cardiomyopathy, but they also show a further increase in velocity higher up in the left ventricle when obstruction is present. In patients who develop a "tunnel" subaortic stenosis secondary to valvular obstruction, increased velocity below the aortic valve can be shown (Figure 6.10).

In patients with fixed subvalvular obstruction, the maximal velocity curve in the ascending aorta is similar to that in valvular stenosis, but if one records with pulsed Doppler from the apex toward the aortic valve, a localized clear increase in velocity below the aortic valve is found in these patients (see Figure 5.20).[6] An example is shown in Figure 5.21. With this method, the presence or development of a subaortic obstruction has been shown also in patients following surgery for complex congenital heart lesions. The localized increase in velocity in subvalvular obstruction differs clearly from the moderately increased velocity that can be seen with increase in flow. In the latter case there is a gradual increase in velocity up through the left ventricle.

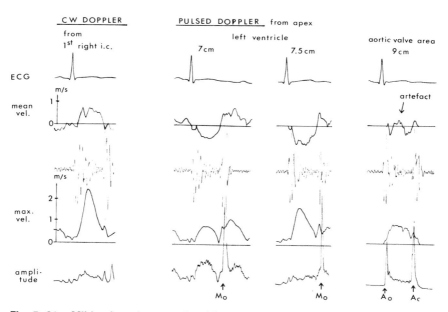

Fig. 5–21. Mild subaortic stenosis with a peak pressure drop of 20 to 25 mm Hg calculated from maximal velocity in the ascending aorta. Pulsed Doppler recording from the apex shows increase in velocity at 7.5 cm depth, 1.5 cm below the aortic valve area. M_o—mitral valve opening; A_c—aortic valve closure; A_o—aortic valve opening.

C. Right Ventricular Outflow Obstruction

In pulmonary valve stenosis, jet velocities can usually be recorded with the transducer in the second or third left intercostal space directed toward the back, slightly upward and medially. Figure 5.22 is from a patient with mild pulmonary stenosis. CW Doppler was first used to find the jet, and then

Doppler Ultrasound in Cardiology

PULMONARY VALVE STENOSIS

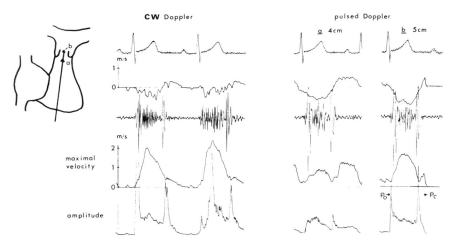

Fig. 5–22.   Pulmonary valve stenosis. With CW Doppler a maximal velocity of 2.4 m/s is recorded, and calculated peak pressure drop is 23 mm Hg. With pulsed Doppler (4cm) a normal velocity is recorded below the pulmonary valve in systole as well as pulmonary valve closure (P$_c$) followed by flow velocity towards the transducer in diastole (pulmonary regurgitation). Increased velocity is recorded at 5 cm depth together with both valve opening (P$_o$) and closure indicating that obstruction is at valve level.

the pulsed mode was used to locate where the increase in velocity occurred, in this case at the valve area.

Figure 5.23 shows that the presence of an obstruction below the valve can be diagnosed. With CW Doppler from the fourth intercostal space, a maximal velocity of 2.5 m/s was recorded. By switching to the pulsed mode a localized increase in velocity exceeding the limits for the pulsed mode was found at 5.5 to 6 cm depth, while the valve area with both the opening and the closing movement of the valve was located 7 cm from the transducer. In infundibular stenosis, the best position and direction to the jet are usually lower and more upward than in valvular stenosis. Figure 5.23 also shows the limitations of both the pulsed and the CW mode if they are used separately and shows how they complement each other when combined (see Section 3.6).

Increased velocity in the pulmonary artery is also seen with increased flow, as in significant left-to-right shunts and with significant pulmonary regurgitation. In these patients, velocity is increased both in the right ventricle and in the pulmonary artery, and there is no marked localized increase as when obstruction is present. An example of increased pulmonary flow velocity in a patient with atrial septal defect is shown in Figure 5.64.

Of 32 patients with signs of obstruction to flow, 19 were correctly diagnosed as valvular stenosis and 13 as infundibular, 7 of the latter had Fallot's tetralogy, and 5 had an associated ventricular septal defect. When both infundibular and valvular stenosis are present as in patients with Fallot's tetralogy, the pulsed mode shows the obstruction at the infundibular level and the continuous mode usually shows the combined pressure drop (unless the direction of the two jets differs too much). Since velocity across even a moderate infundibular obstruction exceeds the limits for the pulsed mode, the presence and degree of an additional valvular obstruction are not possible to assess. With possibilities to record higher velocities in the pulsed mode as described in Chapter 6, such obstructions at two different levels may be separated.

In two of the patients with Fallot's tetralogy, the high-velocity jet in the infundibulum or the pulmonary artery was not found on the first examination, but was recorded at the next one. Both patients were infants with pronounced infundibular obstruction; one also had a hypoplastic pulmonary artery. It is obviously more difficult to detect a long narrow jet in such a case

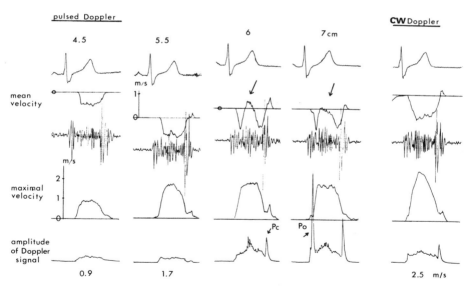

Fig. 5–23. Pulmonary infundibular stenosis. CW Doppler gives a calculated peak pressure drop of 25 mm Hg. With pulsed Doppler, increase in velocity occurs from 4.5 to 5.5 cm, while valve level with valve opening and closure is at 7 cm depth. At 5.5 cm maximal velocity is just within the limit for the pulsed mode; at 6 and 7 cm velocity is higher producing an artifact in the mean velocity curve (reverse deflection in mid-systole marked by arrows).

than to localize a jet in a normal or dilated pulmonary artery where the disturbed flow beside the jet may make it easier to localize the artery.

The question may also be raised whether the pressure drop can be calculated from the maximal velocity using the same formulas as in mitral and aortic stenosis when the length of the obstruction is considerable. So far there has been no indication of underestimation of such obstructions as pressure drops of 60 and 80 mm Hg from the right ventricle to the pulmonary artery have been calculated in two patients one and two days old with Fallot's tetralogy. The patient with a peak pressure drop of 80 mm Hg was later shown to have both pronounced infundibular obstruction and a hypoplastic pulmonary artery.

The diagnosis of infundibular stenosis was missed by Doppler in one patient with a ventricular septal defect and obstruction in the right ventricle because of a transverse muscle band located low in the ventricle. This obstruction caused a high-velocity jet recorded toward the transducer in the third and fourth left intercostal spaces, and was assumed to be caused by the jet through the septal defect which had the same location. Otherwise, the differential diagnosis of ventricular septal defect and infundibular obstruction has not been difficult. The two conditions can usually be separated by finding the different location and direction of the jets (see Figure 5.55). They can be diagnosed also when both lesions are present, except in conditions with equal or near equal pressures in the two ventricles where flow through a septal defect is less likely to be detected. In these conditions, however, the ventricular septal defect is usually easily seen with two-dimensional echocardiography.

Calculated peak pressure drop from the right ventricle to the pulmonary artery in these 32 patients ranged from 12 to 126 mm Hg and correlated well with the peak pressure drop that was recorded at catheterization in 20 of them. It was also possible to assess the degree of pulmonary stenosis in three of four patients with transposition of the great arteries and pulmonary or subpulmonary obstruction where pressure drops of 75 to 113 mm Hg were calculated. The fourth patient in whom signs of obstruction were not recorded had peripheral pulmonary artery stenosis.

The increase in velocity across a banding of the pulmonary artery can be used to assess the degree of obstruction produced. Figure 5.24 is from a two-year-old patient with banding of the pulmonary artery. Increased maximal velocity gave a calculated peak pressure drop of 44 mm Hg and pulsed Doppler showed that increase in velocity and obstruction was 1.5 cm above the pulmonary valve. The increase in splitting of the second heart sound has been used to assess the degree of banding,[14d] but it may not always be easy to determine from the phonocardiogram the timing of P_2. The pulmonary artery flow velocity curve can then be helpful to show the duration of right ventricular ejection. Figure 5.25 is from an infant (10 months) for whom banding of the pulmonary artery was done at two months of age for intrac-

BANDING OF PULMONARY ARTERY

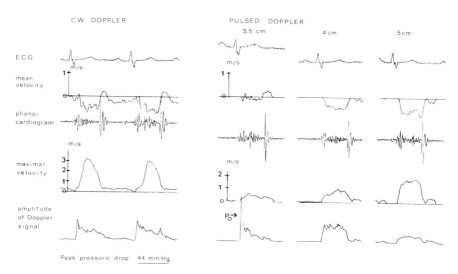

Peak pressure drop   44 mm Hg

Fig. 5–24. With CW Doppler increased velocity is recorded in the pulmonary artery. Pulsed Doppler shows increase in velocity to occur from 4 to 5 cm depth. This is clearly above valve level and shows that the obstruction is located above the valve. Velocity at 3.5 cm is not clearly recorded, most likely due to a large angle to the flow at this level.

table heart failure. A high-velocity jet indicated a tight banding with a calculated peak pressure drop of 85 mm Hg. In addition, in the two to three last beats where the high-velocity jet is lost, the prolongation of right ventricular systole is seen with pulmonary valve closure 70 ms later than A_2.

Following surgery for pulmonary stenosis, assessment of pulmonary valve function has been helpful, especially in patients with associated lesions, a persistent systolic murmur, and right bundle branch block in the electrocardiogram. Of 27 patients seen following surgery (12 with pulmonary stenosis, 14 with Fallot's tetralogy, and one with double outlet right ventricle— DORV), pulmonary regurgitation was present in 20 of them. Several of these, some also with signs of significant regurgitation in the Doppler recording, had no diastolic murmur, only a systolic murmur, even if no residual obstruction was present. The systolic murmur in these patients was probably due to increased flow across the valve from a more than moderate regurgitation.

Of the 12 patients with isolated pulmonary stenosis, six had no residual obstruction and six had an insignificant peak pressure drop of 12 to 20 mm Hg across the valve. Of 14 patients with Fallot's tetralogy, six had no obstruction, and it was insignificant in another five. Three had a residual peak pressure drop of 45 to 46 mm Hg. Two of them were operated upon as infants

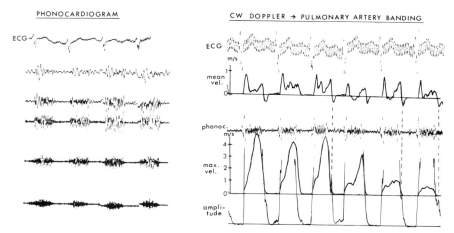

Fig. 5–25. A CW Doppler recording of flow velocity in the pulmonary artery in a 10-month-old child. Banding of the pulmonary artery was done at the age of two months. Maximal velocity was 4.6 m/s with a calculated peak pressure drop of 85 mm Hg. Peak pressure drop occurs late in systole indicating a late maximum of right ventricular systolic pressure (this can only be judged in the first beat, not in the others owing to loss of part of the signal in systole). The timing of the pulmonary valve closure was not easy to identify in the phonocardiogram, but the velocity and ampli- tude curves show that flow continues well beyond A$_2$ and that pulmonary valve closure is much later (stippled line). With a gradual decrease in gain, fewer of the high velocities in the signal are recorded. Note that the duration of the amplitude is the same as that of the maximal velocity and that the latter continues beyond A2 even with a minimal gain setting. This shows that the high velocity is not an artifact caused by a gain setting that is too high or a Doppler signal that is too strong (see Figs. 5.81 and 5.82).

because of severe symptoms. These findings agreed with the results of a postoperative catheterization performed in 12 of the 27 patients.

Since only three of the 27 patients had a clear residual obstruction, the systolic murmur present in many of them was therefore more frequently caused by the presence of regurgitation with increased flow across the valve than by residual obstruction.

Similar results were found in another hemodynamic study following oper- ation for pulmonary valve stenosis.[14e]

Pulsed Doppler has been used to detect the presence of pulmonary ste- nosis or right ventricular outflow obstruction from disturbed flow in the pulmonary artery or right ventricular outflow tract,[14f, 9] but this gives only the diagnosis and not the degree of obstruction.

D. Tricuspid Valve Stenosis

The presence of tricuspid stenosis is easy to diagnose with Doppler. The transducer is directed to the right from a position at the left sternal border or more toward the apex, depending on the size of the right ventricle. Velocities as high as in mitral stenosis are not found, but the Doppler signal is clearly different from that of normal tricuspid flow. Velocities are moderately increased, but they decrease slowly during diastole. Increases with inspiration are more pronounced than in normal subjects. When significant tricuspid regurgitation is present, foward tricuspid flow velocity may also be increased, but the increase is then of shorter duration.

In Figure 5.26 velocity of tricuspid flow in a normal subject is shown together with the increased velocity due to regurgitation in one patient and to tricuspid stenosis in another. From the maximal velocity recorded, a pressure drop may be calculated as in other obstructions, and seems so far to correlate well with pressure drop obtained by catheter withdrawal from the right ventricle to the right atrium. An example is shown in Figure 5.27 where the variation in maximal velocity and calculated pressure drop with respiration can be seen. The patient had a moderate tricuspid stenosis following de Vega's annuloplasty. At catheterization a mean pressure drop of 3 mm Hg across the tricuspid valve was found. In another patient a mean pressure drop of 5 to 7 mm Hg was recorded with Doppler following tricuspid repair. Similar pressure drops have been reported from invasive studies in a larger group of patients following repair of tricuspid regurgitation.[15] Tricuspid stenosis has also been recorded in some patients with a long history of rheumatic mitral valve disease, some of them with earlier mitral valve replacement. Calculated mean pressure drops in these patients were from 3 to 6 mm Hg. The clinical diagnosis of tricuspid stenosis had not been suspected previously in any. Figure 5.28 shows a recording from a patient with mild mitral and tricuspid stenosis, while Figure 5.29 is from a patient with mitral valve prosthesis and rheumatic tricuspid stenosis.

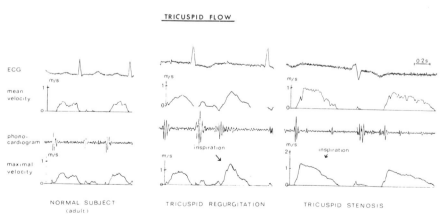

TRICUSPID FLOW

Fig. 5–26. Pulsed Doppler recording of tricuspid flow velocity. The increase in velocity recorded in the patient with tricuspid stenosis is moderate, but is clearly different from normal and from the increase in forward flow velocity in tricuspid regurgitation.

TRICUSPID VALVE STENOSIS

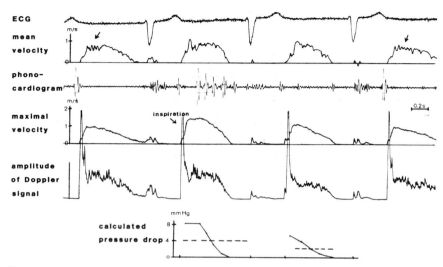

Fig. 5–27. Pulsed Doppler recording of tricuspid valve stenosis following de Vega's annuloplasty. Maximal velocity of tricuspid flow is increased throughout most of diastole despite a slow heart rate (48 beats / min). The increased frequency shift with inspiration is easily heard, and the second beat shows the clear increase in maximal velocity and calculated pressure drop. Indentations in the mean velocity curve (arrows) were caused by flutter of the tricuspid valve early in diastole.

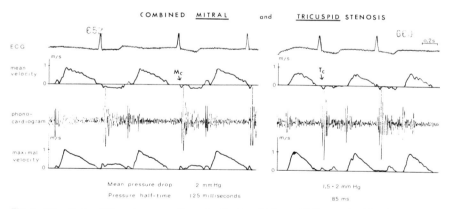

Fig. 5–28. Pulsed Doppler recording of mitral and tricuspid flow velocities in a patient with both mild mitral and tricuspid stenosis. The velocity curves are quite similar in this case, but tricuspid flow starts earlier in relation to the second heart sound, and decrease in velocity is slightly more rapid. Tricuspid flow starts earlier and closure of the tricuspid valve (T_c) is later than the mitral (M_c).

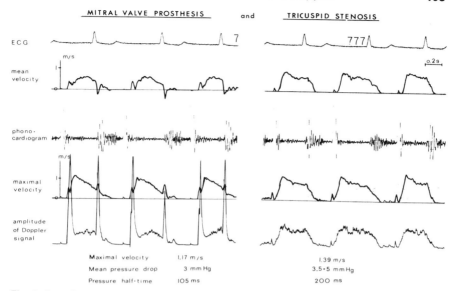

Fig. 5–29. Pulsed Doppler recording showing the mild obstruction to flow through a normally functioning mitral valve prosthesis (Björk-Shiley) and the moderate flow obstruction at the tricuspid valve in the same patient. The strong reflections from the prosthetic valve are seen in the amplitude curve.

When one is recording velocity of tricuspid flow, it is not easy to overlook the presence of tricuspid stenosis, and the diagnosis was rapidly made in the seven patients seen so far. This is in contrast to catheterization where the diagnosis, especially in atrial fibrillation, may be more difficult owing to the changes with respiration, unless right atrial and ventricular pressures are recorded simultaneously.

5.3   VALVE REGURGITATIONS

A.   Aortic Regurgitation

The presence of aortic regurgitation can be shown, by recording with pulsed Doppler from the apex, as flow velocity toward the transducer below the aortic valve in diastole, or from the suprasternal notch as reverse flow velocity in diastole in the ascending or descending aorta. Figure 5.30 shows the mean velocity in the ascending aorta with flow toward the transducer in systole and away from the transducer throughout diastole (A). In the descending aorta, the same pattern but with opposite direction is found (B). When one is recording from the apex, the aortic valve is first localized, and the area just below the valve is then searched for regurgitant flow velocity with the pulsed mode. Regurgitation starts at aortic valve closure and continues throughout diastole (C). The quality of the Doppler signal from aortic

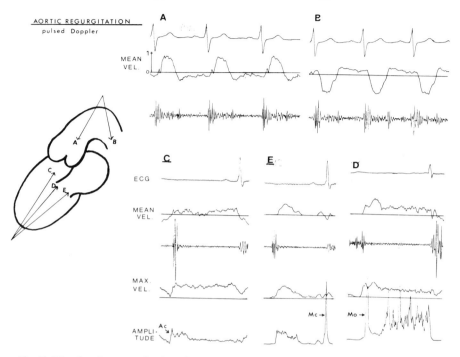

Fig. 5–30.   Aortic regurgitation. A and B show reverse flow velocity in diastole in the ascending and descending aorta. C shows regurgitation recorded just below the aortic valve. It starts at aortic valve closure (A$_c$). E, Close to the mitral valve area only forward mitral flow velocity is recorded with mitral valve closure (M$_c$). D, In a position between C and E, fluttering of the mitral valve is present throughout diastole and best recorded in the amplitude curve. Aortic regurgitation is seen before mitral valve opening (M$_o$).

regurgitation is quite different from that of mitral flow which is also toward the transducer in diastole. The two flow velocity patterns can also be separated by recording the regurgitation high in the left ventricular outflow tract (C) and mitral flow velocity close to the mitral valve (E), as shown in Figure 5.30. In positions between C and E, velocities from both aortic regurgitation and mitral flow are usually present in the sample volume. Aortic regurgitation can then be seen to start before mitral valve opening (D). In positions where the mitral valve opening is recorded, fluttering of the mitral valve is easily heard as frequently repeated valve movements throughout diastole, and is best seen in the amplitude curve (D). It differs clearly from the mitral valve flutter found in conditions with increased flow across the mitral valve or in flail mitral leaflet where the flutter is mainly found during rapid filling (early diastole and following atrial contraction).

The diagnosis of aortic regurgitation is best made by recording with pulsed Doppler just below the aortic valve where even very small degrees can easily be recorded. In the ascending or descending aorta, moderate to severe degrees of regurgitation can easily be shown, but small degrees can be overlooked. One must also be aware of other conditions that may cause reverse diastolic flow in the descending aorta (patent ductus arteriosus, aorticopulmonary or aorticosubclavian shunts). Since the pressure difference between the aorta and the left ventricle in diastole is significant, high velocities in aortic regurgitation may be recorded with CW Doppler from the apex. Figure 5.31 is from a patient with combined aortic stenosis and regurgitation. The high velocities in the regurgitation are seen to decrease during diastole as the aortic left ventricular pressure difference decreases.

The detection of aortic regurgitation with Doppler from the suprasternal notch as well as from the left ventricle has been described.[16,16a,b] The diagnosis is easy also when mitral stenosis is present. This has been found by other investigators as well.[16c]

Figure 5.32 is from a patient with isolated aortic regurgitation recorded from the apex with CW Doppler. The Doppler signal contained both high and many low frequencies, indicating a position to the side of the jet or a

AORTIC STENOSIS AND REGURGITATION

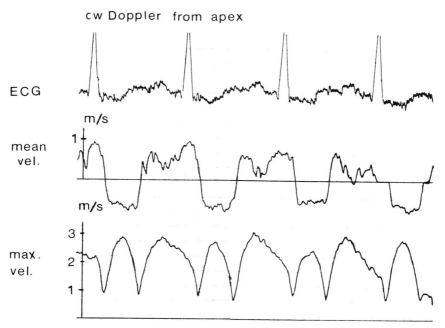

Fig. 5–31. CW Doppler recording from apex towards the aortic valve shows increased maximal velocity in systole due to aortic valve stenosis, but also shows that high velocities are present in the regurgitation. Maximal velocity in the regurgitation decreases during diastole as the pressure difference between aorta and left ventricle decreases.

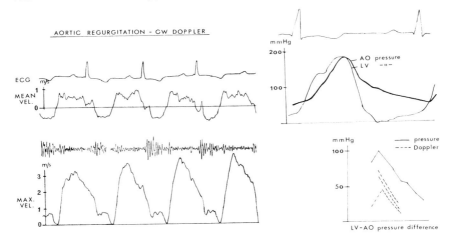

Fig. 5–32. **Maximal velocities in aortic regurgitation recorded from apex with CW Doppler. The Doppler signal was mixed with both high and low velocities. Comparison between calculated and recorded aortic left ventricular diastolic pressure difference also indicates that a substantial angle between ultrasound beam and regurgitant jet has been present.**

substantial angle. Comparison with pressure recording shows that maximal velocity and aortic left ventricular pressure drop in diastole are underestimated. With a good Doppler signal, a rapid decrease in maximal velocity to a low velocity at end-diastole indicates a large regurgitation with near equalization of pressures. Even if high velocities are frequently recorded in aortic regurgitation, a signal with mainly high frequencies is not as frequently found and a calculated aortic left ventricular pressure drop, therefore, is often unreliable. If velocity is still high at end-diastole (see Figure 6.10), however, it shows that aortic and left ventricular pressures are far from equalized.

The degree of aortic regurgitation may be assessed from the relation between forward and reverse flow velocities in the aorta. Good results have been reported with CW Doppler directed toward the aortic arch / descending aorta[16,17] or pulsed Doppler in the ascending or descending aorta.[18,19,19a] The latter would be expected to be better since venous flow velocities during diastole may be recorded with CW Doppler. Pulsed Doppler recording of reverse diastolic flow velocities in the subclavian arteries has been found useful by some.[20,21] A better flow signal can often be obtained from a subclavian artery than from the ascending aorta as illustrated with the spectral analysis in Figure 5.33, but a Doppler with a higher frequency must be used to record from the more superficial vessel. Reversed diastolic flow velocity in the subclavian arteries may also be seen in patent ductus arteriosus when blood flow is from the systemic circulation to the pulmonary artery, and then it is more pronounced in the left than the right subclavian artery. Some reverse flow in diastole can often be recorded in the subclavian arteries in

AORTIC REGURGITATION

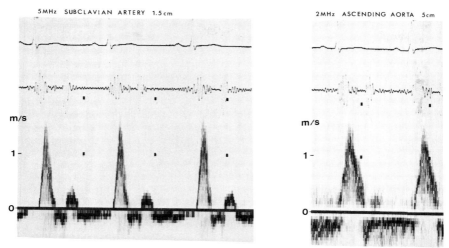

Fig. 5–33. In aortic regurgitation a better flow velocity signal can usually be obtained from a subclavian artery than from the aorta, and with spectral analysis a more narrow band of frequencies is seen.

normal individuals, and the flow velocity pattern may change rapidly, presumably by changes in peripheral resistance (e.g., by changes in room temperature).[21a,b]

B. Pulmonary Regurgitation

Pulmonary regurgitation is diagnosed in a similar way by recording at and below the pulmonary valve with pulsed Doppler. Figure 5.34 is from a patient with pulmonary regurgitation following operation for Fallot's tetralogy. The regurgitant flow toward the transducer in diastole is best recorded below the pulmonary valve, but was in this case recorded also above valve level (7 cm). This is usually seen when more than moderate degrees of regurgitation are present. The degree of regurgitation can also be assessed from the extension into the right ventricle and probably from the intensity of the Doppler signal. With significant regurgitation, a moderately increased velocity in the right ventricle and the pulmonary artery in systole can be found. In the patient in Figure 5.34, all these features were present, indicating that the regurgitation was more than moderate. When large regurgitations are present, there may be no diastolic murmur, but there is a prominent third heart sound at the lower left sternal border simultaneously with peak velocity of the regurgitation.

Figure 5.35 is from a patient with pulmonary regurgitation secondary to pulmonary hypertension. Regurgitation was recorded throughout diastole below the valve, but was not recorded at or above the valve level. The

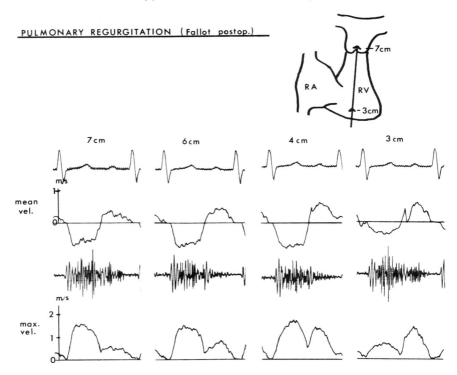

Fig. 5–34. Pulsed Doppler recording of flow velocity in the right ventricle (3 to 6 cm) and in the pulmonary artery (7 cm) in a patient operated on for Fallot's tetralogy. Regurgitation is toward the transducer in diastole. It is best recorded below the valve, but is also recorded above. The velocity of the regurgitation decreases rapidly and ends before systole indicating that a pressure drop is no longer present between pulmonary artery and the right ventricle at end-diastole.

regurgitation could not be recorded in the lower part of the right ventricle and the intensity of the Doppler signal from the regurgitation was low, both indicating a moderate degree of regurgitation. That regurgitation continues throughout diastole only shows that a pressure drop between the pulmonary artery and the right ventricle is still present at end-diastole. In contrast, the velocity of the regurgitant flow in Figure 5.34 decreases rapidly and ends before systole indicating equalization of pressures in the right ventricle and pulmonary artery at end-diastole. With high diastolic pressure in the pulmonary artery, velocity in the regurgitation jet is high and can be recorded with CW Doppler if a reasonable angle can be obtained and if the amount of regurgitation is not too small. With a Doppler signal with mainly high frequencies, a diastolic pulmonary artery-right ventricular pressure difference may be calculated, or if maximal velocity is still high at end-diastole, it indicates raised diastolic pulmonary artery pressure.

The form of the velocity curve in the pulmonary artery in Figure 5.34 is rounded as normal, whereas in Figure 5.35 an early peak, followed by early decrease in maximal velocity, is seen. This change in the velocity curve is probably due to increased pulmonary vascular resistance since it is regularly found in patients with clearly increased resistance.[22]

Diastolic flutter of the tricuspid valve is found in some patients with significant regurgitation, but not as regularly as in aortic regurgitation. With pulsed Doppler, the presence of pulmonary regurgitation has been shown in several patients, especially those with pulmonary hypertension where a diastolic murmur was not heard.

In normal subjects, flow velocity toward the transducer in diastole can sometimes be recorded just below the pulmonary valve. This flow signal is usually easily lost with small changes in depth or the direction of the beam, and it may be difficult to record consistently throughout diastole. It is usually recorded when the beam is aimed laterally and anteriorly in relation to the valve area, and this may represent flow in the anterior descending branch of

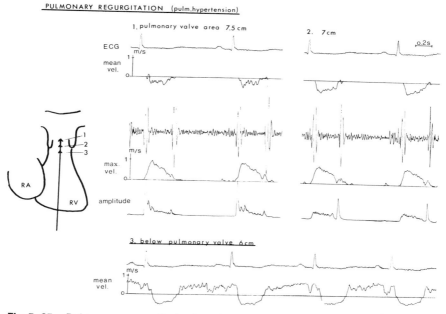

Fig. 5–35. Pulmonary regurgitation in pulmonary hypertension recorded with pulsed Doppler. Flow velocity toward the transducer is found below the valve during diastole, but is not recorded at valve level or above. Regurgitation continuing throughout diastole shows that a pressure difference is still present between the pulmonary artery and the right ventricle at end-diastole. Pulmonary valve closure is early, and the early peak velocity of flow in pulmonary artery is characteristic of pulmonary hypertension with increased resistance to flow. Mean velocity at valve area is not clearly recorded because of systolic fluttering of the pulmonary valve.

the left coronary artery recorded simultaneously with flow at the pulmonary valve area. Figure 5.36 shows such a recording from a healthy child. The flow toward the transducer starts in early diastole and velocity decreases during diastole. This pattern is quite similar to that reported earlier with a Doppler ultrasonic catheter flow meter in the left or right coronary artery.[23] This flow velocity signal may be mistaken for pulmonary regurgitation. Clues in the differentiation are the very limited area where it can be recorded, as well as a more anterior and lateral direction in relation to the valve area (realized when scanning the pulmonary valve area). The best differentiation probably is that this is a flow signal that sounds normal with a narrow band of frequencies and that signs of disturbed flow with more and lower frequencies cannot be shown. A similar clear signal may occasionally be obtained from a regurgitant jet, but a slight change in direction then also gives the signs of disturbed flow beside the jet. Pulmonary regurgitation can usually be recorded further down in the right ventricle and more medially and posteriorly in relation to the valve area as indicated in Figure 5.36. If one changes to a smaller probe, these two normal flow velocity patterns may no longer be recorded simultaneously in contrast to pulmonary flow and regurgitation.

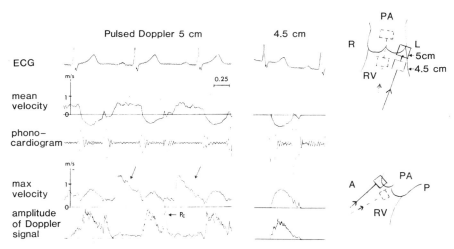

Fig. 5–36. Flow velocity patterns recorded in the right ventricle just below the pulmonary valve in a healthy subject. (Pc—pulmonary valve closure). Flow is away from the transducer in systole. At 5 cm depth also, flow toward the transducer is recorded during most of diastole. This flow velocity signal could only be recorded at this depth. It was easily lost with only slight movements of the transducer and with chest movements during respiration indicating a narrow blood flow. It was recorded fairly laterally and anteriorly (unbroken line) compared to the area where flow velocity toward the pulmonary artery and pulmonary valve movements could be recorded. As suggested in the drawing, this flow pattern may represent blood flow in the descending branch of the left coronary artery. A slightly more medial direction was necessary to get a good flow velocity signal from the pulmonary artery (stippled line). Pulmonary regurgitation is usually recorded at a more central position (stippled line) and over a larger area. A—anterior; P—posterior; R—right; L—left.

C. Tricuspid Regurgitation

If one records from the apex or the left sternal border, tricuspid regurgitation is diagnosed when reverse velocity of flow occurs at the tricuspid orifice and can be followed back into the right atrium. Several directions of the ultrasound beam at the tricuspid orifice should be attempted since the regurgitant flow may have a different direction than forward tricuspid flow. Regurgitation is usually detected easily using either the pulsed mode at the tricuspid orifice or the continuous mode toward the right atrium.

Figure 5.37 shows a recording of tricuspid regurgitation with pulsed and CW Doppler. In the right ventricle (RV) at 5 cm depth (pulsed Doppler), only forward diastolic flow velocity is recorded. The variation with respiration is clearly seen. Close to the tricuspid orifice (7 cm), tricuspid valve opening and closure are recorded as well, and in the orifice (8 cm) both forward diastolic and reverse systolic flow velocity are recorded together with valve movements which show lower amplitude at this level. The reverse systolic flow velocity can also be recorded further back in the right atrium (RA—9 cm). The regurgitation starts at the tricuspid valve closure and continues past the second heart sound until tricuspid valve opening.

Maximal velocity in the regurgitation recorded with pulsed Doppler is about 1 m/s, which is the limit for the pulsed mode at this depth. The mean velocity curve shows two nearly positive peaks (8 cm) which indicates that higher velocities are present than those recorded with the pulsed mode. Switching to the continuous mode shows a maximal velocity of 3.5 m/s in the tricuspid regurgitation from an angle where the highest frequency shift in the jet was found. From this maximal velocity, a pressure drop can be calculated as in the presence of obstructions. The recorded velocity of 3.5 m/s gives a calculated pressure difference of 49 mm Hg from RV to RA in systole. Maximal velocity in the tricuspid regurgitation can therefore be used to assess RV systolic pressure. With too large an angle between the ultrasound beam and the regurgitant jet, maximal velocity and the pressure drop are underestimated. The tricuspid regurgitation is usually easy to find and comparison between pressure drop calculated from maximal velocity and pressure drop obtained at catheterization has shown good correlation.[24] This indicates that small angles to the regurgitant jet can usually be obtained. If RV pressure is high, but the amount of regurgitation is small, there are high frequencies in the Doppler signal, but with low intensity. The low intensity gives an inferior signal/noise ratio, and it may be difficult or impossible to record these high frequencies even if they are heard in the audio signal. With moderate or larger degrees of tricuspid regurgitation, however, the high frequencies are usually easily recorded, making possible calculation of RV-RA pressure difference in systole.

The degree of regurgitation can be roughly assessed. When regurgitation is significant, it can be recorded further back in the right atrium, intensity of the Doppler signal is higher, and velocity of forward flow through the tricuspid valve is increased.[24] When a large regurgitation is present, this can be

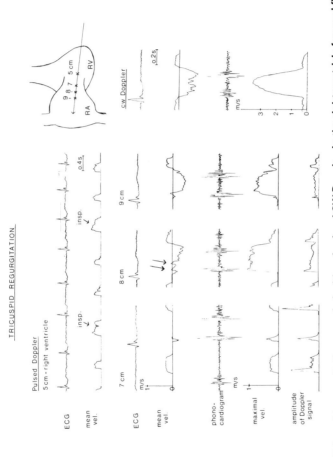

Fig. 5–37. **Tricuspid regurgitation recorded with pulsed and CW Doppler. In the right ventricle forward flow velocity in diastole increasing with inspiration is recorded. Close to the orifice (7 cm), valve movements are also recorded. At 8 cm both forward diastolic and reverse systolic flow velocities are present and valve movements are less clearly recorded. Arrows point to artifacts in the mean velocity curve caused by the presence of velocities above the limit for the pulsed mode. CW Doppler shows a maximal velocity of 3.5 m/s, with a calculated RV-RA pressure drop at 49 mm Hg in systole. RV systolic pressure is, therefore, 50 to 55 mm Hg (or higher if maximal velocity is underestimated).**

recorded not only in the orifice and the right atrium, but also in the right ventricle. In Figure 5.38, flow away from the transducer in systole is clearly recorded at 4.5 and 5 cm where normally only forward diastolic flow and perhaps some systolic flow toward the transducer would be recorded. The reverse systolic flow velocity can be followed back into the right atrium. This pattern is usually seen in Ebstein's malformation, but also in other cases where regurgitation is severe. The Doppler signal from such large regurgitations may sound like normal blood flow without signs of disturbed flow. This may be because of a large area of regurgitation as well as a low RV-RA pressure difference in systole.

Tricuspid regurgitation with Doppler has been diagnosed from measurements of venous flow velocity curves[25] and by recording in the right atrium with pulsed Doppler combined with M-mode[26] or two-dimensional echocardiography.[27]

Validation of the diagnosis of tricuspid regurgitation with Doppler has been clearly shown by Stevenson, et al.[27a] Doppler is a sensitive method for

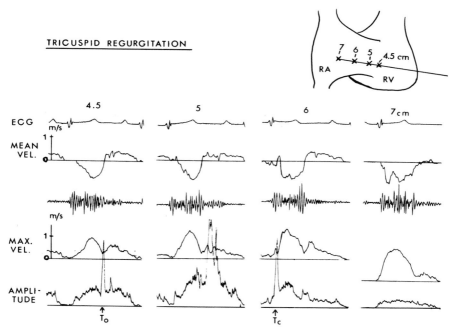

Fig. 5–38. When regurgitation is large, reverse systolic flow may also be recorded in the right ventricle (RV). With pulsed Doppler, the regurgitant flow velocity in this patient was recorded almost as well in the right ventricle as in the atrium. In normal individuals flow velocity in the RV in systole is toward the transducer if recorded close to the tricuspid orifice. At 5 cm diastolic flutter of the tricuspid valve was present due to the increased flow across the valve. T_o—tricuspid valve opening; T_c— tricuspid valve closure.

diagnosis of tricuspid regurgitation and has shown the low sensitivity of the clinical diagnosis.[24] The presence of tricuspid regurgitation can also be demonstrated by contrast echocardiography and M-mode recording from the inferior venae cava,[27b,c] but Doppler is a more sensitive method when the regurgitation is mild or moderate.[27d] Since microbubbles are easily detected with Doppler, use of Doppler instead of M-mode to detect contrast in the inferior vena cava might improve the sensitivity.[27e] Since the regurgitation in mild cases, however, may be recorded only a short distance behind the valve, recording in the vena cava is still likely to be less sensitive.

Quantification of the regurgitation has also been attempted 1) by recording the extension of disturbed flow in the right atrium and the inferior vena cava,[27f] 2) by showing the extension of reverse flow in the right atrium with a multigated Doppler and color-coding showing the direction of flow,[27g] and 3) by comparing reverse and forward flow in the inferior vena cava.[27h]

D. Mitral Regurgitation

The presence of mitral regurgitation can be shown by recording from the apex with pulsed Doppler at the mitral valve area and behind the valve in the left atrium. Figure 5.39 shows at 9 cm depth both forward diastolic and reverse systolic flow velocity as well as the opening and closing movement of the mitral valve. Forward flow velocity is less than at 7 cm. At 10 cm, forward flow and valve movements are barely recorded while regurgitation is clearly present. This regurgitant flow velocity is not recorded in the left ventricle. The negative flow velocity in systole at 7 cm depth is from flow toward the aorta. The systolic flow velocity in the left ventricle starts after the first heart sound and ends at aortic valve closure in contrast to the mitral regurgitation which starts earlier at mitral valve closure and continues past the second heart sound until mitral valve opening. The main difference, however, lies in the quality of the Doppler signal. The normal systolic flow in the left ventricle is tone-like with few frequencies. In mitral regurgitation many different, mostly low frequencies are heard when recording with pulsed Doppler; with CW Doppler, recording from the jet gives mainly very high frequencies, and beside the jet mainly various low frequencies.

With CW Doppler from the apex, it is usually easy to detect the abnormal Doppler signal from mitral regurgitation in systole. The high frequencies may, however, have low intensity and be more difficult to record than in tricuspid regurgitation, possibly because of a longer distance from the transducer. Figure 5.40 shows recording of mitral regurgitation with CW Doppler. A maximal velocity of 4 m/s gives a calculated peak pressure drop of 64 mm Hg from the left ventricle to the left atrium. Even with moderately increased left ventricular systolic pressures, velocities up to the limit for the applied Doppler may be recorded (6 m/s ~ a pressure drop of 144 mm Hg). The CW mode also shows the negative velocities in systole more clearly than the pulsed mode where the mean velocity curve may be disturbed by artifacts.

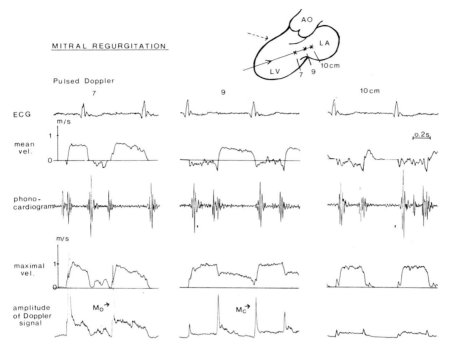

Fig. 5–39. **Mitral regurgitation recorded with pulsed Doppler from apex. When the sample volume is moved toward the left atrium, regurgitation is recorded at the valve area at 9 cm depth. The negative systolic flow velocity recorded at 7 cm is from normal systolic flow in the left ventricle. Mitral regurgitation starts earlier and lasts until mitral valve opening. The maximal velocity curve of forward mitral flow shows that a moderate mitral stenosis is also present. M$_o$—mitral valve opening; M$_c$—mitral valve closure.**

When mitral regurgitation is detected with CW Doppler, this may not always be possible to confirm with pulsed Doppler as described, since patients with large hearts may have a mitral valve area that is 12 cm or more from the apex (maximal depth for the pulsed mode). A more parasternal position of the transducer may then be used to diagnose the regurgitation even if this may increase the angle to the regurgitant jet (Figure 5.39, stippled arrow). Another method of showing that an abnormal systolic flow velocity recorded with CW Doppler is due to mitral regurgitation is to make use of the range ambiguity of the pulsed mode. Figure 5.41 illustrates that a flow velocity signal at a certain depth also can be recorded a shorter distance from the transducer (depth − 8 cm). If the valve area at 9 cm were located at 12 cm depth instead, only the forward diastolic flow velocity would be recorded, but the sequence of forward diastolic to reverse systolic flow velocity shown from 8 to 11 cm in Figure 5.41 would then be located at 12 to 15 cm and it could then be recorded at 4 to 7 cm depth. The use of this range

MITRAL REGURGITATION, CW Doppler

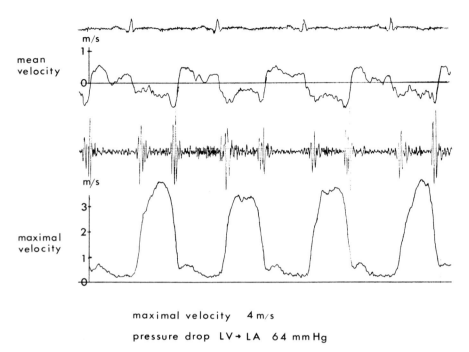

mean
velocity

maximal
velocity

maximal velocity   4 m/s

pressure drop LV → LA   64 mm Hg

Fig. 5–40.   Mitral regurgitation recorded with CW Doppler from the apex.

ambiguity to diagnose mitral regurgitation is helpful in patients with large hearts, since the Doppler signal, in the continuous mode, from the regurgitation may in this group show low intensity and sometimes be difficult to record.

In the presence of significant mitral regurgitation, velocity of forward mitral flow is often increased. When regurgitation causes an increased V-wave in the left atrial pressure curve, left atrial-left ventricular pressure difference early in diastole is higher than normal and maximal velocity of forward flow therefore is increased. Since the pressures equalize rapidly, this increase in velocity is of short duration in contrast to the increase in velocity caused by obstruction at the valve. In a few patients with significant regurgitation, a clear increase in early diastolic flow velocity is not seen. These are patients with large atria where even a large regurgitation may be present without increased left atrial pressure.[28]

Flail mitral leaflet is easily diagnosed with pulsed Doppler as shown in Figure 5.42. The pronounced flutter of parts of the mitral valve during filling

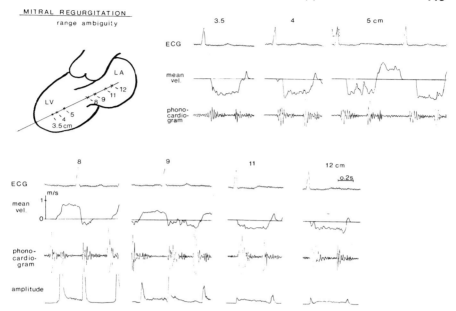

Fig. 5–41. Pulsed Doppler recording of mitral regurgitation. Regurgitation is recorded from the valve area from 9 cm to 12 cm. Because of the range ambiguity of the pulsed mode, the same velocity signal can also be recorded with a depth setting of 8 cm less than where the velocity occurs. In this case no Doppler signal was recorded less than 3.5 cm from the transducer. From 3.5 to 5 cm mitral regurgitation is recorded (actually at 11.5 to 13 cm). At 5 cm both the forward mitral flow at 5 cm and the regurgitation at 13 cm are recorded. This range ambiguity can be used to diagnose mitral regurgitation when the mitral valve area is 12 cm or more from the transducer.

periods in the left ventricle and at the valve area or behind in the left atrium throughout systole is easily heard. The strong signals from the fluttering valve may disturb recording of the flow velocity at the valve area, but in these cases mitral regurgitation is usually so large that the reverse flow in systole also can be recorded 1 or 2 cm into the left ventricle.

When both mitral and tricuspid regurgitation are present in the same patient, they can be separated by the different location and direction of the regurgitant jets, by the difference in forward flow velocity curves, and by the different timing of valve opening and closure of the two A-V valves. Figure 5.43 is from a patient with both mitral and tricuspid regurgitation and shows the difference in timing of the valve movements. The tricuspid valve closes later than the mitral as normal, but in this case also opens later as it is delayed by the presence of pulmonary hypertension.[29-30] Mitral valve opening is earlier due to mitral stenosis.

The diagnosis of mitral regurgitation with pulsed Doppler combined with M-mode[19,31-33,33a,b] and with 2D-echocardiography[34-35,35a] has been de-

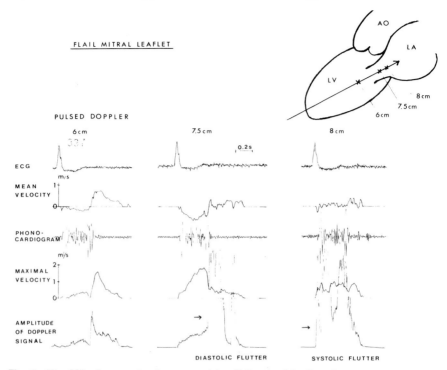

Fig. 5–42.   Mitral regurgitation caused by flail mitral leaflet. At 6 cm mitral valve opening and increased velocity of forward flow are recorded, while velocity in systole comes from normal left ventricular flow. At 7.5 cm the mitral valve flutter during diastolic filling is prominent and velocity of flow, therefore, is less clearly recorded. The negative velocity in systole comes from mitral regurgitation. (The Doppler signal in systole is abnormal at this depth. Flow also starts at the beginning of the first heart sound and continues until mitral valve opening.) Mitral valve closure is recorded at 8 cm and is followed by pronounced systolic flutter of the valve which disturbs the recording of flow velocity.

scribed, and a high degree of specificity and sensitivity reported. A false positive diagnosis was described in one patient with increased flow in the left atrium in systole due to anemia. This should not occur when one is recording in a direction toward the mitral orifice and detecting the regurgitant flow velocity at the orifice as described here, instead of the transverse direction usually applied in M-mode echocardiography. With M-mode the method was found to be less sensitive in patients with mild regurgitation, mitral valve prolapse, or a cleft mitral valve.[33a,b] With the technique of recording the regurgitation in the orifice and into the left atrium this has not been a problem, but in such cases the regurgitation sometimes could be recorded only 1 to 2 cm behind the valve. This may explain the inferior sensitivity with

Doppler combined with M-mode, and the combination with 2D-echocardiography might improve the sensitivity in such cases.

The degree of mitral regurgitation may be assessed as described for tricuspid regurgitation by the extension of the regurgitation in the left atrium, by the intensity of the Doppler signal from the regurgitation, and from increases in forward flow velocity. Experience so far indicates that this is usually possible. Assessment of the degree of mitral regurgitation from the aortic flow velocity curve recorded with Doppler has been described.[36] With significant mitral regurgitation, aortic flow velocity decreases earlier in systole. A similar aortic flow velocity pattern with the major part of forward flow velocity recorded during the first part of systole is usually seen also in patients with hypertrophic obstructive cardiomyopathy. Assessment of the degree of regurgitation from only the extension in the left atrium compared well with the assessment from left ventricular angiograms in one study.[33]

5.4 PROSTHETIC VALVES

The slight or moderate obstruction to flow caused by most prosthetic valves results in increased velocity of flow across the prosthesis, and a

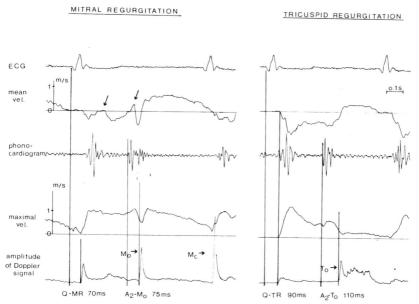

Fig. 5–43. Pulsed Doppler recording of mitral and tricuspid regurgitation in one patient. The difference in timing of start of regurgitation and valve openings is shown. Velocity of forward mitral flow shows that mitral stenosis is present as well. Arrows indicate artifacts in mean velocity curve due to presence of high velocities in the mitral regurgitation.

pressure drop can be calculated from the increase in velocity as in valve stenosis. Holen, et al. found that in mitral valve prostheses a pressure drop obtained from velocity recordings correlated well with a pressure drop recorded at catheterization.[37] In most patients velocity curves from flow across mitral valve prostheses can be recorded as easily as in mitral stenosis. It may take longer to find the best position and direction with disc valves where flow depends on the orientation of the valve and the direction of the major opening. As in mitral stenosis, velocity and pressure drop, in addition to valve area, depend on heart rate and flow across the valve, cardiac output, as well as eventual regurgitant flow. Pressure half-times are slightly longer than across normal valves ($<$ 60 ms), usually between 70 and 120 ms, varying with type and size of prosthesis. Figure 5.29 shows the flow velocity recorded across a normally functioning disc valve in the mitral position.

Figure 5.44 shows velocity of flow across another mitral valve prosthesis (Hancock, size 27). The velocity curves are similar to those obtained in mild mitral stenosis. Calculated mean pressure drop was 6 mm Hg; at catheterization a mean pressure drop of 7 mm Hg was found. Pressure half-time was 120 ms, slightly prolonged as in mild obstruction. Doppler recording during bicycling in the supine position showed an immediate increase in velocity. A mean pressure drop of 12 mm Hg at a heart rate of 95, increasing to 20

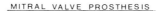

MITRAL VALVE PROSTHESIS

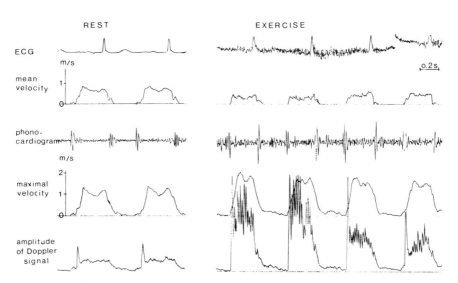

Fig. 5–44. Flow velocity across a mitral valve prosthesis (Hancock) at rest (pulsed Doppler) and during exercise (CW Doppler). Calculated mean pressure drop at rest is 6 mm Hg and during exercise 12 mm Hg at a heart rate of 95. During exercise pronounced fluttering of the prosthetic valve occurred.

mm Hg at a heart rate of 110, was calculated. These results are in the range reported from hemodynamic studies for this prosthesis.[38] With exercise and increased velocity across the prosthesis, pronounced fluttering of the valve occurred, which is shown in the amplitude curve in Figure 5.44. It was not present at rest and disappeared shortly after exercise. Diastolic flutter of porcine mitral valves shown with M-mode echocardiography has been described in aortic regurgitation, and diastolic and systolic flutter has been described in torn and flail porcine valves.[39] The diastolic flutter recorded in this patient only on exercise indicates that increased flow or a high velocity through the prosthesis may cause the fluttering. This might also be the cause of the diastolic flutter reported in one patient with paravalvular leakage.[40] In the patient shown here there was no sign of regurgitation, which is usually easy to detect with Doppler in porcine valves. Similar pressure drops have been recorded also in other tissue valves (Carpentier-Edwards prosthetic valve).

Figure 5.45 is from two different patients. To the left, high maximal velocities are recorded throughout diastole and give a calculated mean pressure

MITRAL VALVE PROSTHESIS

increased pressure drop caused by:

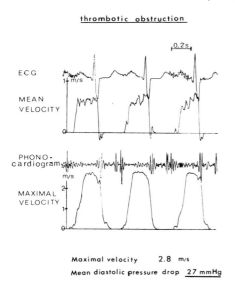
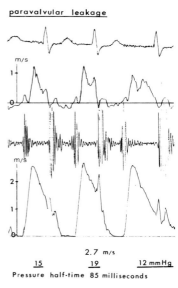

Fig. 5–45. Increased maximal velocity and pressure drop across mitral valve prosthesis. In the patient to the left, the high velocity is sustained throughout diastole indicating that obstruction causes the increased pressure drop, whereas to the right the high velocity decreases rapidly indicating that significant obstruction is not present. In the latter, the increased velocity may be caused by increased flow across the prosthesis.

drop of 27 mm Hg. The patient was in pulmonary edema and with CW Doppler, the diagnosis of severe obstruction at the mitral valve could be made within a minute. In the patient to the right in Figure 5.45, a maximal velocity in the same range as in the first patient was recorded, but velocity decreased rapidly during diastole. Pressure half-time was only slightly longer than normal but not longer than usual for this prosthesis (Bjørk-Shiley prosthetic valve, size 31), indicating that obstruction of the prosthesis was not present. With the high maximal velocity recorded and short diastole, the mean pressure drop across the valve was still significant. Increased flow across the prosthesis is, therefore, the likely explanation for the increased velocity. Increased flow may be due to either increased cardiac output or leakage beside or through the prosthesis. With high cardiac output, high velocities in the ascending aorta or across other valves would be expected, whereas with significant mitral regurgitation, aortic flow velocity is usually reduced or at least not high. To record regurgitant flow velocity directly through the prosthesis, as in mitral regurgitation, is not easy with disc valves since Doppler signals from behind the prosthesis are difficult to obtain. Recording beside the prosthesis may be done, but makes orientation uncertain without the aid of echocardiography. Paravalvular leakage may, however, be shown more easily, as the regurgitant jet may, in such cases, be easier to reach. With tissue valves, regurgitation can be shown as well as with ordinary valve regurgitations. Figure 5.46 shows obstruction and regurgitation in a tricuspid valve prosthesis. Regurgitation is demonstrated by recording with pulsed Doppler in the right ventricle, through the prosthesis, and into the right atrium. Velocity of forward flow is significantly increased and the sustained high velocity in diastole indicates that this is due not only to increased flow across the prosthesis, but to additional obstruction as well.

Although regurgitation in mitral valve prosthesis is usually difficult to record, regurgitation in aortic valve prosthesis is easily recorded in the left ventricle below the prosthesis. Semiquantitation is possible, as in aortic regurgitation. Good Doppler signals from the ascending aorta can be obtained in some patients with aortic valve prosthesis, whereas it may be difficult in others. It is usually easy in those patients in whom good Doppler signals from the aortic jet can be recorded before the operation. The best position is usually the first or second right intercostal space as in aortic valve stenosis. Figure 5.47 shows four patients with aortic valve prosthesis. Increased maximal velocity with a calculated peak pressure drop above that recorded across normal aortic valves[8] was found in all. The result in the patient with a Bjørk-Shiley valve is close to that reported from hemodynamic studies[41] where the mean pressure drop was 19 mm Hg in a patient with this valve size. In the third patient shown in this figure, a pressure drop of 15 mm Hg across the prosthesis was recorded at catheterization when the heart rate was 70, whereas at the ultrasonic examination the heart rate was 47 (complete heart block) and stroke volume and pressure drop were presumably higher.

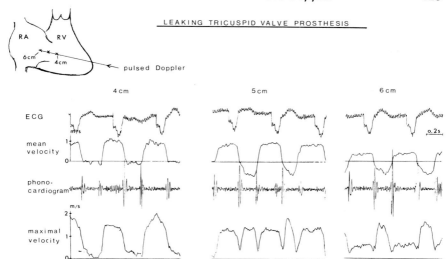

Fig. 5–46. Obstruction and regurgitation in tricuspid valve prosthesis (Hancock) recorded with pulsed Doppler. The increased maximal velocity of forward flow gives a calculated mean pressure drop of 8 to 10 mm Hg across the prosthesis. At 5 cm depth both opening and closing movements of the prosthetic valve were recorded (not shown here) as well as regurgitant flow velocity during systole. At 6 cm forward flow velocity is reduced while regurgitation is still clearly recorded.

AORTIC VALVE PROSTHESES

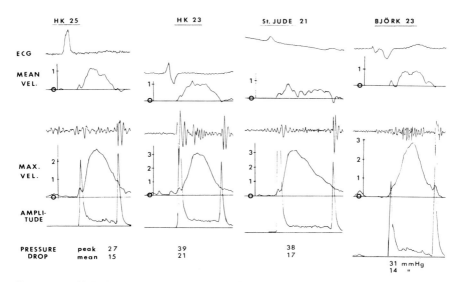

Fig. 5–47. Velocities recorded with CW Doppler in the ascending aorta in four patients with aortic valve prostheses. HK—Hall-Kaster; Bjørk—Bjørk-Shiley.

In Figure 5.48, maximal velocity in the ascending aorta gives a calculated peak and mean pressure drop of 30 and 11 mm Hg. In this case an increase in velocity was recorded in the left ventricle 2 cm below the aortic prosthesis where a subvalvular membrane had been removed at operation. At the valve level, repeated frequent movements of the prosthetic valve during systole were heard. The moderate pressure drop may, therefore, be partly due to a slight residual subvalvular obstruction and partly to the prosthetic valve (Hall-Kaster, size 23).

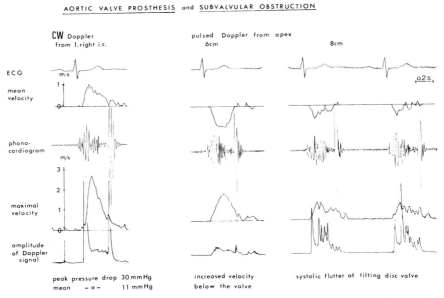

Fig. 5–48.   Increased maximal velocity recorded in the ascending aorta in a patient with aortic valve prosthesis. With pulsed Doppler from apex increased velocity is recorded 2 cm below the prosthetic valve, and systolic fluttering of the valve is present. The increased velocity in the ascending aorta could therefore be partly due to the prosthesis and partly due to a residual subvalvular obstruction.

5.5   HYPERTROPHIC CARDIOMYOPATHY (HCM)

In hypertrophic cardiomyopathy, changes in flow velocity patterns can be found both in the left ventricle and in the ascending aorta in systole and in the mitral flow velocity curve in diastole.

A.   Flow Velocity in the Left Ventricle

When obstruction to flow occurs, increased velocities are present in the left ventricle, and a high-velocity jet away from the transducer in systole can be recorded with CW Doppler from the apex. The direction of this high-velocity jet is usually toward the mitral orifice or is slightly more medial and superior, but is not quite as high as toward the aortic valve, except when a subaortic tunnel is present. If there is no mitral regurgitation, an intraventricular pressure can be calculated from the maximal velocity recorded. Figure 5.49 is recorded from a patient in whom mitral regurgitation was not found either with Doppler or on left ventricular angiography. Pulsed Doppler showed increase in velocity in the left ventricle and since there was no mitral regurgitation, the high velocity recorded with CW Doppler could be assumed to be in the left ventricle.

HOCM   cw Doppler from apex

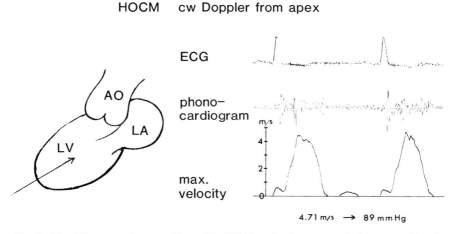

4.71 m/s → 89 mm Hg

Fig. 5–49. When one is recording with CW Doppler from apex in hypertrophic obstructive cardiomyopathy (HOCM), a high velocity jet away from the transducer in systole can be found (mean velocity showing direction of velocity not included here). Direction of the ultrasonic beam is usually toward the mitral orifice or slightly higher, but below the aortic valve area. In diastole, mitral flow velocity (toward the transducer) is recorded. In this patient mitral regurgitation was not present, allowing calculation of an intraventricular pressure drop from the maximal velocity recorded. With pulsed Doppler, increase in velocity was recorded at 7 cm depth while mitral and aortic valve area was found 11 and 12 cm from the transducer.

When mitral regurgitation is present, a high-velocity jet away from the transducer in systole and in the direction of the mitral valve is found with CW Doppler. The directions of the jet caused by the obstruction in the left ventricle and by the mitral regurgitation may, therefore, be similar. They may only be possible to separate when obstruction is high in the left ventricular outflow tract with a clearly more superior direction of the increased velocity from the obstruction. In patients with mitral regurgitation, an intraventricular pressure drop cannot usually be calculated from a CW Doppler recording. The diagnosis of an intraventricular obstruction in addition to mitral regurgitation can still be made by pulsed Doppler. Figure 5.50 shows increase in

HYPERTROPHIC OBSTRUCTIVE CARDIOMYOPATHY

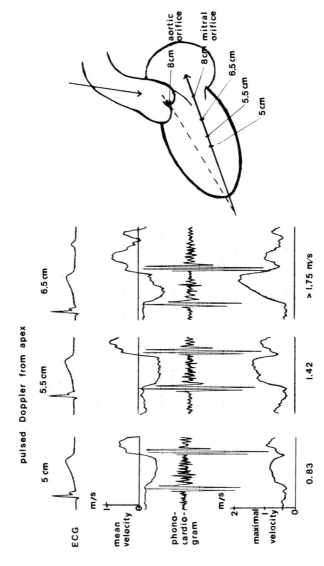

Fig. 5.–50.   Pulsed Doppler recording in the left ventricle in HOCM. Increased velocity is recorded at 5.5 cm depth in a direction toward the mitral orifice at 8 cm depth. The transducer had to be directed more upward to record the aortic valve. Arrow in ascending aorta shows beam direction when recording from the suprasternal notch indicating that the high velocity in the left ventricle in this condition is not usually recorded with CW Doppler from above because of the large angle between ultrasound beam and velocity.

128

velocity recorded within the left ventricle in a patient with HCM. Since 1.75 m/s is the limit for the pulsed mode within 7.5 cm depth, a pressure drop above 10 to 15 mm Hg cannot be shown with pulsed Doppler. Since most patients with hypertrophic obstructive cardiomyopathy (HOCM) have mitral regurgitation, comparison between pressure drop calculated from CW Doppler recording of maximal velocity and pressure drop recorded at catheterization have so far been possible in too few patients to know if a maximal velocity comparable to the pressure drop present can usually be recorded. So far, however, the presence of an intraventricular pressure drop has been diagnosed in all patients when it has been present at catheterization.

With a higher pulse repetition rate, higher velocities can be recorded in the pulsed mode. A higher pressure drop in the left ventricle can then be shown also when mitral regurgitation is present. However, with higher pulse repetition rates, problems with range ambiguity increase (see Section 3.3B and Figure 3.7) as the distance between two successive pulses easily becomes less than the distance to the signal to be recorded. Figure 5.51 shows how the flow velocity signals from the left ventricle in a patient with HCM also can be recorded closer to the transducer than where it occurs (the previous pulse being picked up at the shorter distance). This range ambiguity may present problems in depth localization of recorded signals, but may also be of advantage since recording a signal closer to the transducer than at the depth where it occurs allows a higher velocity to be recorded in the pulsed mode. In this case 2.15 m/s was recorded at 6 cm depth, while at the ambiguous depth a velocity of 2.45 m/s could be recorded. Increased velocities earlier in systole and above this level were not recorded in this patient. This is described in more detail in Chapter 6.

The flow velocity curve where increase in velocity is first recorded (closest to the transducer) often shows a late systolic maximum, as depicted in Figures 5.51 and 5.52. This increase occurs later in systole than the decrease in the aortic flow velocity curve (see Figure 5.52) assumed to be caused by obstruction, and it may be followed by an abrupt decrease in velocity or cessation of flow before end-systole. This pattern is found below the level of the mitral valve and most likely corresponds to the near emptying of the apical portion of the left ventricle that can be seen with two-dimensional echocardiography and on angiograms. Above this level, flow disturbances may be recorded earlier in systole, but high velocities cannot usually be shown due to a larger distance to the transducer.

Even if the obstruction is more than 7.5 cm from the transducer and increased velocities cannot be shown in the pulsed mode, a signal of disturbed flow with many low frequencies of high intensity can be used to localize the obstruction from mid-ventricular obstruction to higher in the left ventricular outflow tract. In the latter position the sound of valve movements may be heard in mid-systole coinciding in time with the anterior systolic

HYPERTROPHIC OBSTRUCTIVE CARDIOMYOPATHY

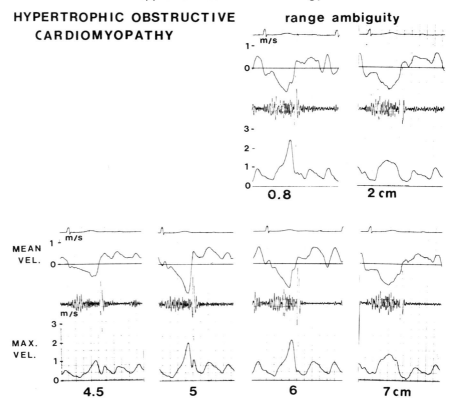

Fig. 5–51. When a pulsed Doppler with a higher pulse repetition rate is used, a maximal velocity of 2.15 m/s is recorded at 6 cm depth. The same flow velocity signal can also be recorded 5.2 cm closer to the transducer, and at this depth a velocity of 2.45 m/s is recorded.

movement of the mitral valve recorded on echocardiograms immediately before or after the Doppler recording. At the aortic valve area, the systolic fluttering of the aortic valve can be clearly heard.

B. Flow Velocity in the Ascending Aorta

Figure 5.52 also shows a flow velocity curve from the ascending aorta recorded with pulsed Doppler from the suprasternal notch. Peak velocity is early, before onset of the systolic murmur, and is followed by a more rapid decrease than normal. In the second half of the prolonged systole, only low velocities are recorded. The start of the decrease in flow velocity usually coincides with the start of the systolic murmur, while the late systolic increase in velocity low in the left ventricle occurs later, starting at peak murmur.

HYPERTROPHIC OBSTRUCTIVE CARDIOMYOPATHY

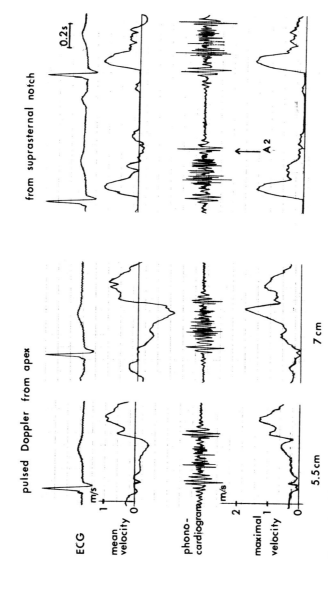

Fig. 5-52. A late systolic increase in velocity in the left ventricle recorded with pulsed Doppler. In the ascending aorta peak velocity is early before onset of murmur, and is followed by a sharp decrease. In the second half of the prolonged systole, only low velocities are recorded.

131

Increased velocities in the ascending aorta, as in valvular or fixed subvalvular obstruction, are not usually recorded either with pulsed or CW Doppler in patients with HCM. With CW Doppler some of the high velocities present in the left ventricle might be recorded also from the suprasternal notch, but the distance to the increased velocity is larger and, as indicated in Figure 5.50, the angle to this velocity is usually too large.

A change in the aortic flow velocity curve in HOCM was first described by estimating velocity from recorded pressure drop[42] and from flow velocity recording during operation.[43] A noninvasive diagnosis of the abnormal flow velocity pattern was made by recording from the carotid artery with a 5 MHz CW Doppler and later from the descending aorta with a 2.2 MHz CW Doppler.[44, 45] When recording from the carotid artery was done, the pattern with early and sharp decrease in velocity was noted only in patients with HOCM and was not observed in a large group of patients with a variety of other conditions.

The disturbed flow within the left ventricle has been recorded with pulsed Doppler.[34, 46] Murgo, et al. have recently described the flow velocity pattern in the ascending aorta recorded with electromagnetic catheter flow meter as well as the rate of ejection of blood from left ventricular angiograms in patients with HCM.[47] They found a flow velocity pattern that differed significantly from normal with a larger amount of blood ejected early in systole in patients both with and without obstruction, indicating that a more rapid ejection of blood, and not necessarily obstruction, may lead to the observed flow velocity curve.

Figure 5.53 shows a flow velocity curve from the ascending aorta in one patient with obstruction and in another without obstruction together with a

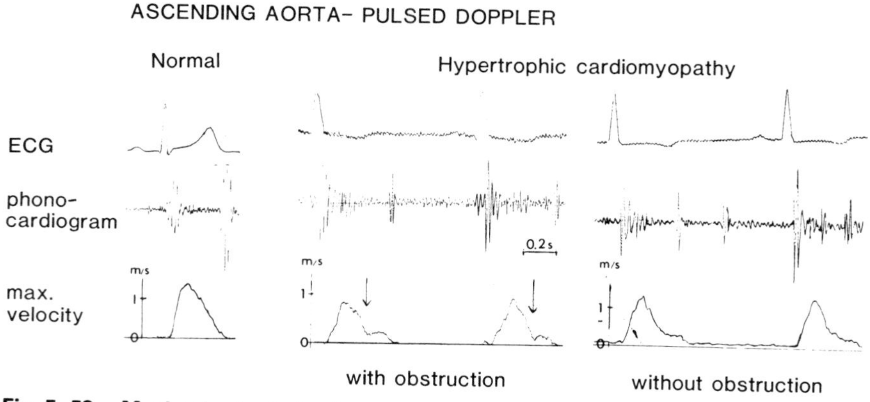

ASCENDING AORTA- PULSED DOPPLER

Fig. 5–53. Maximal velocity in the ascending aorta in a normal subject compared to the velocity recorded in a patient with HOCM and in one with hypertrophic cardiomyopathy without obstruction. A similar change is seen in both the patient with and without obstruction with more of the flow velocity recorded early in systole. Systole is prolonged in the patient with obstruction (LVETc 459 ms).

curve from a normal subject. In both patients with HCM, most of the flow velocity is recorded in the first half of systole, and a more rapid decrease in velocity in mid-systole is seen also in the patient without obstruction. Left ventricular ejection time is prolonged in the patient with obstruction (LVETc 459 ms) and is normal in the one without obstruction (LVETc 400 ms). Similar flow velocity curves have been recorded in many other patients with HCM in both the presence and the absence of obstruction; these are comparable to the results obtained with electromagnetic flow meters and angiography.[47]

Significant mitral regurgitation may also cause a change in the aortic flow velocity curve with a larger part of the stroke volume ejected during the first half of systole.[36] In significant mitral regurgitation, a shortened LVET would be expected, whereas in HCM a normal or prolonged LVET has been found whether mitral regurgitation has been present or not. Murgo, et al. found no significant difference in the aortic flow velocity curves in HCM between patients with or without mitral regurgitation.[47]

C. Mitral Flow Velocity

The mitral flow velocity curve differs from normal in most patients with HCM. Maximal velocity in early diastole is usually normal, but the decrease that follows is in most patients slower than normal (see Figure 5.51). If a pressure half-time is calculated as in mitral stenosis, a slightly prolonged one is found in most: 60 to 120 ms compared to less than 60 ms in normal subjects and 100 to 400 ms in mitral stenosis. In a few patients, a mitral flow velocity curve indistinguishable from that recorded in mitral stenosis can be found, with both increased maximal velocity and more prolonged pressure half-time. In these patients, either mitral valve calcifications with reduced valve opening or severe hypertrophy in the inflow region restricting valve opening have been present on two-dimensional echo. The more moderately delayed decrease in velocity seen in the majority is often combined with increased velocity following atrial contraction. These patterns are seen also in other patients with left ventricular hypertrophy and nondilated ventricles as in aortic stenosis. In Figure 5.73 (Section 5.7C), these changes are compared to a normal mitral flow velocity curve.

The increase in velocity at atrial contraction may be caused by increased late diastolic filling or by a more forceful atrial contraction due to increased resistance to filling.[48] The slower decrease in velocity or slightly prolonged pressure half-time indicates a slower equalization of left atrial and ventricular pressures than normal, which could be due to a prolonged relaxation. Similar mitral flow velocity curves in left ventricular hypertrophy have also been reported by others.[48a] The relaxation process has been shown to extend into diastole both in animals[49] and in man.[50] Echocardiographic studies have also indicated slower early diastole filling,[51, 52] and abnormal or prolonged relaxation in patients with HCM or with left ventricular hypertrophy from pressure overload.[52, 53] The reduced rate of decrease in flow velocity can be compared to the reduced EF slope seen on M-mode,[54] but with Doppler the lack of increase in maximal velocity makes possible a distinction between decreased filling due to hypertrophy and to mitral stenosis (as discussed in Section 5.2A).

5.6 CONGENITAL HEART LESIONS

A. Ventricular Septal Defect (VSD)

Ventricular septal defects have been diagnosed with high sensitivity and specificity using combined pulsed Doppler and M-mode echocardiography.[32, 55-56] The diagnosis was made by recording a Doppler signal of disturbed flow in the right ventricle in systole and following this into and through the septum, thereby also localizing the defect. The direction of the shunt, the pulmonary vascular resistance, and the localization of the VSD influenced the ability to diagnose the defect. Problems have included differentiation of left ventricular right atrial shunts from VSD endocardial cushion defects and differentiation between supracristal defects and right ventricular outflow obstruction. The presence of additional shunts or valvular regurgitations was easily diagnosed.

With CW and pulsed Doppler, without simultaneous echocardiography, experience has been somewhat similar. VSD with a left-to-right shunt and with a clear pressure drop from the left to the right ventricle has been diagnosed easily. Patients with inlet defects, patients with mainly right-to-left shunts, and patients with large VSDs and right ventricular pressure close to or equal to that of the left ventricle have been difficult to diagnose. In some newborns or young infants with large but otherwise uncomplicated VSD and without a systolic murmur, the VSD could not be diagnosed by Doppler until weeks later when a murmur was present. Then a jet into the right ventricle could be easily shown and a pressure drop calculated from the left to the right ventricle. In these children the defect is usually large enough to be easily shown with two-dimensional echocardiography.

When a left-to-right shunt is present, the diagnosis of VSD with Doppler alone can be made by recording a high-velocity jet into the right ventricle in systole. The area of the right ventricle is scanned with CW Doppler to detect abnormal flow signals and, if these signals are present, pulsed Doppler is used to locate them within the right ventricle. The continuous mode is then used to try to obtain a small angle to the direction of the jet. If the direction of the jet as indicated by the CW mode and the localization with the pulsed mode are combined, the defect can be localized high or low in the septum, close to the aortic and/or tricuspid valve, or in the right ventricular outflow tract.

In Figure 5.54 a maximal velocity of 4.7 m/s was recorded with CW Doppler from the third left intercostal space, giving a calculated pressure

VSD - CW Doppler

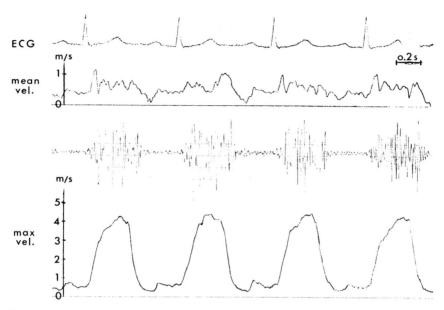

Fig. 5–54. Maximal velocity in VSD jet recorded with CW Doppler. Velocity toward the transducer in diastole is from tricuspid flow. A maximal velocity of 4.7 m/s gives a left-to-right ventricular pressure drop of 88 mm Hg.

drop of 88 mm Hg between the left and the right ventricle. With a systolic blood pressure of 120 mm Hg, this indicates a right ventricular systolic pressure of less than 32 mm Hg. Pulsed Doppler showed that the velocity of blood flow started early in systole and was directed toward the transducer at a depth of 2 to 4 cm. Since tricuspid flow velocity was present in the sample volume, this flow signal had to be located in the right ventricle.

With the variable direction of the jet in relation to the chest wall with different localizations of the defects, different positions and directions should be tried to obtain a small angle to the jet, usually from the second to the fourth left intercostal spaces. When small angles and high velocities are obtained, left to right ventricular pressure drop can be calculated and low or normal right ventricular pressures estimated. In a study of 75 patients with VSD, a high pressure drop across the VSD could be shown in about half the patients where this was present.[57] If only low velocities are recorded, this may be due to either a large angle to the jet or a high right ventricular systolic pressure. Estimations of systolic pulmonary artery pressure from the pulmonary valve closure-tricuspid valve opening interval can then be helpful.[29, 30, 57] In a few patients with VSD and a large left-to-right ventricular pressure drop, the low frequencies in the Doppler signal may be of so high intensity that high velocities are difficult to record. This is further discussed in Section 5.9. Spectral analysis improves the recording of high-velocity jets in these patients (see Chap. 6).

The differentiation between right ventricular outflow obstruction and VSD located in that part of the ventricle can be made by finding the direction of the abnormal flow velocity recorded. The direction of the jet in infundibular pulmonary stenosis is upward and can be followed into the pulmonary artery while direction of the VSD jet is more forward. Even when both are present, they can usually be separated by recording two different jets with different directions. Figure 5.55 is from an adult with a subpulmonary VSD. Recording toward the VSD allowed the pulmonary valve closure to be heard, but the transducer had to be aimed more superiorly to record the pulmonary valve properly. The best directions for recording flow at the pulmonary valve area (away from the transducer) and through the VSD (toward the transducer) are indicated by the arrows in Figure 5.55. Apart from the difference in direction, flow through the VSD can be shown to start earlier than flow into the pulmonary artery. The difference is usually around 20 ms, but longer in the

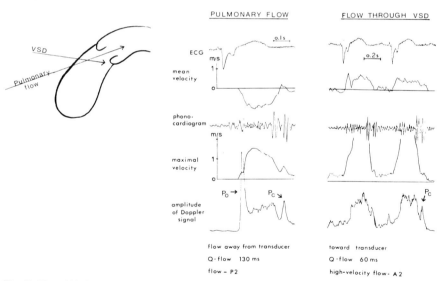

Fig. 5–55. **CW Doppler recording of flow velocity into the pulmonary artery as well as into the right ventricular outflow tract through a ventricular septal defect (VSD). The difference in transducer directions to record the two velocity curves is indicated by the arrows. Velocity of flow through the VSD is toward the transducer whereas flow velocity into the pulmonary artery is away from the transducer. Pulmonary valve closure (P$_c$) was recorded together with flow velocity through the VSD indicating that the latter was located shortly below the pulmonary valve. The start of flow into the pulmonary artery, which is much later than through the VSD, is partly due to a right bundle branch block present in this patient.**

patient in Figure 5.55 due to right bundle branch block. Maximal velocity recorded through the VSD was 4.6 m/s, which is not shown with the scale used in the figure. In patients with Fallot's tetralogy, the presence of a VSD in addition to right ventricular outflow obstruction can sometimes be shown, but not in all patients, owing to similar right and left ventricular pressures.

In patients with acute myocardial infarction in whom a pansystolic murmur and sudden deterioration develop, Doppler has been useful in differentiating between septal rupture and mitral regurgitation due to rupture of a papillary muscle. Of seven such patients, VSD was diagnosed easily in four and severe mitral regurgitation in the three others. Diagnosis of VSD in acute myocardial infarction has been described also with pulsed Doppler combined with M-mode echocardiography.[58]

B. Patent Ductus Arteriosus (PDA)

In patent ductus arteriosus with lower resistance in the pulmonary than the systemic circulation, blood flows from the aorta into the pulmonary artery in both systole and diastole (Figure 5.56). In diastole the shunt flow comes from both the ascending and descending aorta as well as the subclavian arteries. This causes reverse diastolic flow, except in the ascending aorta where forward diastolic flow velocity may be more clearly recorded than usual. Reverse diastolic flow velocity in the descending aorta and subclavian arteries can be recorded also in aortic regurgitation and in aorticopulmonary windows or shunts. The conditions can be distinguished by pulsed Doppler recorded at different depths in the ascending and descending aorta to find where the reversal of diastolic flow velocity starts.

Figure 5.57 is from a patient with patent ductus arteriosus. In the ascending and first part of the descending aorta, forward flow velocity only was recorded. At 5 cm depth, a change in the audio signal was noted with signs of disturbed flow during diastole. Recording 1 cm further down in the descending aorta demonstrated reversal of flow velocity in diastole. In subclavian pulmonary artery shunts, a somewhat similar picture can be seen with reversal of diastolic flow in the descending but not ascending aorta. However, an area with signs of disturbed flow at the level of the ductus is not found.

With this approach, the presence of a patent ductus arteriosus has been shown in adults, children, and infants. Following surgical closure, normal flow velocity patterns have been recorded.

The presence of a patent ductus arteriosus with left-to-right shunt can also be shown by recording flow velocity in the pulmonary artery from the left sternal border (Figure 5.58). At the level of the pulmonary valve, valve movements and flow away from the transducer in systole and possibly during atrial contraction are found. Diastolic flutter of the pulmonary valve is sometimes recorded, presumably caused by the jet through the duct reaching the valve. Systolic flutter may also be recorded, but this is found in other condi-

Aortic flow in patent ductus arteriosus

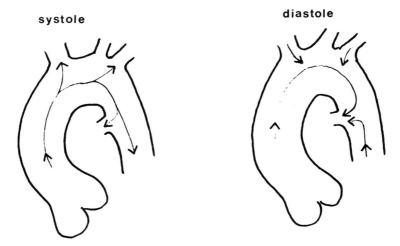

systole   diastole

Aortico-pulmonary shunt

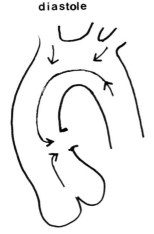

diastole

Aortic regurgitation

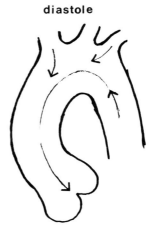

diastole

Fig. 5–56. Reverse diastolic flow in the descending aorta and in the subclavian arteries can be found in aortic regurgitation as well as in aorticopulmonary shunts and
patent ductus arteriosus with left-to-right shunts. The conditions can be distinguished
by recording with pulsed Doppler at different sites in the ascending and descending
aorta.

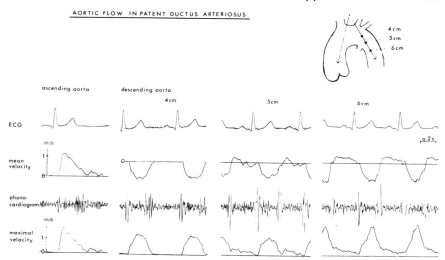

AORTIC FLOW IN PATENT DUCTUS ARTERIOSUS

Fig. 5–57. Pulsed Doppler recording of flow velocity in the ascending and descending aorta. At 5 cm depth, a disturbed flow velocity signal during diastole was noted in the descending aorta. Distal to this area reverse diastolic flow velocity was recorded, while above this area and in the ascending aorta only forward flow velocity was present. The slight increase in maximal velocity in systole at 6 cm depth was due to an insignificant coarctation.

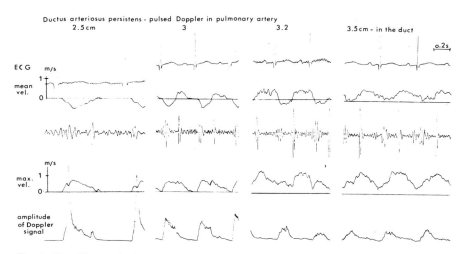

Ductus arteriosus persistens - pulsed Doppler in pulmonary artery

Fig. 5–58. Flow velocity in pulmonary artery in patent ductus arteriosus. At valve level only flow away from the transducer is recorded. Above valve level, flow toward the transducer in diastole is found, and in the duct continuous flow toward the transducer.

tions as well as in normal individuals. By recording further up in the main pulmonary artery, 1 cm or more depending on the size of the patient, one can record flow toward the transducer in diastole. Sometimes flow velocity in the duct itself is recorded (see Figure 5.58, at 3.5 cm) and is toward the transducer in both systole and diastole when the shunt is only from left to right. The flow velocity toward the transducer in the pulmonary artery usually continues throughout diastole, but a shorter duration when increased pulmonary vascular resistance is present has been described.[59] Figure 5.59 is from a patient with pulmonary artery pressure and vascular resistance at systemic level. Flow velocity into the pulmonary artery from the duct was recorded in late systole and first part of diastole. The velocity curve at valve level (3 cm) shows an earlier peak than usual, a pattern seen when pulmo-

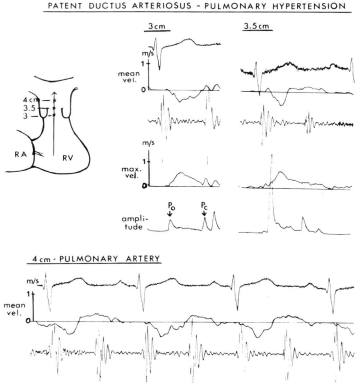

Fig. 5–59. In this patient with patent ductus arteriosus and pulmonary artery pressure at systemic levels, flow through the duct into the pulmonary artery is recorded only in late systole and early diastole. At 3 cm depth only, flow away from the transducer is recorded. Pulmonary valve opening (P_o) and closure (P_c) indicates that this is at the valve area. At 3.5 cm, flow toward the transducer in late systole and early diastole appears, and this is also recorded at 4 cm where valve movements are no longer heard.

nary vascular resistance is increased. In patients with severe pulmonary hypertension from other causes, reversal of flow in the pulmonary artery in late systole can be found. This ends, however, with the second heart sound, whereas flow through the patent duct continues longer into diastole. The Doppler signal also differs, indicating disturbed flow in the patent duct, but not with the reversed flow in pulmonary hypertension.

Usually the presence of a patent ductus arteriosus can be shown both in the descending aorta and in the pulmonary artery, but if coarctation of the aorta is also present, the velocity pattern in the descending aorta changes and the presence of a patent ductus can be shown only by recording in the pulmonary artery. Care must be taken while recording both in the aorta and the pulmonary artery to obtain a central position in the vessel so that simultaneous recording from the artery and nearby veins is avoided. This can be done by listening to the audio signal while slight changes in transducer direction are made. Reversal of flow in more peripheral arteries, such as the brachial arteries, has also been described.[60] It is usually easily recorded in the subclavian arteries. More reversal of flow can be seen on the left than on the right side.

The recording of patent ductus arteriosus in the pulmonary artery with the precordial approach and a combined pulsed Doppler and M-mode has been reported to be both sensitive and specific,[60a] while recording in the right pulmonary artery from the suprasternal notch was found useful to detect or exclude systemic to pulmonary communications.[60a, b]

The degree of reverse flow velocity in the descending aorta may give some indication of the amount of left-to-right shunting, but represents only part of the diastolic flow into the pulmonary artery. Shunting during systole is not easy to assess. With a large left-to-right shunt, increased velocity across the mitral valve can be recorded, but this is useful only in the absence of associated defects.

Patency of the ductus arteriosus has been shown also in premature infants as small as 900 g. In these patients, recording in the pulmonary artery is usually the most useful approach. A 4 or 5 MHz Doppler is easier to apply, but the 2 MHz Doppler can be used from the subcostal position to increase the distance to the pulmonary artery. In small infants, a combined Doppler and echo is probably easier to use and has been found helpful.[60c, d]

Figure 5.60, which is from a patient with an aorticopulmonary shunt, shows how this can be differentiated from patent ductus arteriosus and aortic regurgitation. Reversed diastolic flow velocity is recorded in both the ascending and descending aorta, but not just above the aortic valve, or in the left ventricle (not shown in figure).

With subclavian to pulmonary artery shunts, reversed diastolic flow is recorded in the descending aorta, whereas in the ascending aorta forward diastolic flow is increased. This is similar to findings in patent ductus arteriosus, except that an area of disturbed flow in the aortic arch is not found,

Ultrasonic recording of aortic flow in aorticopulmonary shunt

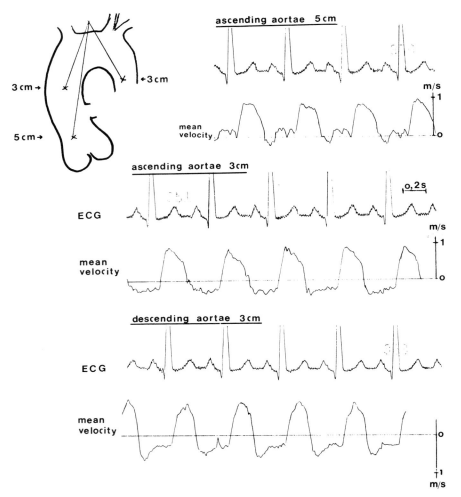

Fig. 5–60. **Pulsed Doppler recording of aortic flow velocity in a patient with an aorticopulmonary shunt shows reverse diastolic flow velocity in both the descending and ascending aorta except in the first 2 cm above the aortic valve.**

possibly because of the different location of these outlets from the aortic arch.

C.   Coarctation of the Aorta

In coarctation of the aorta, pulsed Doppler recording shows signs of disturbed flow at the level of and below the coarctation. With CW Doppler, a high-velocity jet from beyond the coarctation may be recorded. This is usually easily found in patients with a moderate coarctation. With more pronounced coarctation, the jet is found in about 50% of the cases. The difficulties in these patients are probably caused by eccentric localization of the orifice and the jet. When a high-velocity jet has been found, the recorded maximal velocity has given a calculated pressure drop in the same range or a little higher than when systolic blood pressures in the arm and the thigh are compared. The calculated pressure drop may be higher since this drop represents the peak pressure drop in systole. The blood pressure differences are between peak pressures above and below the coarctation. These pressure peaks do not occur simultaneously. The peak pressure below the coarctation occurs later.

Figure 5.61 is from a patient with a moderate coarctation. Abnormal flow velocity signals and increased velocity were recorded at a depth of 6 cm from the suprasternal notch. Arrows point to artifacts in the mean velocity curve. These are not present with the CW mode, which shows a maximal velocity of 3.6 m/s. Calculated peak pressure drop is 52 mm Hg, while systolic blood pressure in the arm is 130 mm Hg and in the thigh 60 to 70 mm Hg.

D. Atrial Septal Defect (ASD)

With pulsed Doppler and M-mode echocardiography, a certain flow velocity pattern has been shown in the right atrium in ASD with left-to-right shunt. Flow has been toward the transducer starting in early or mid-systole, increasing toward end-systole and with a second increase during atrial con-

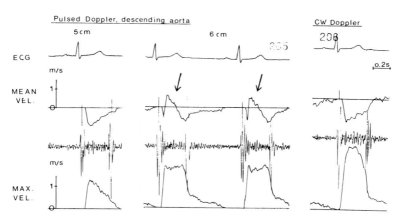

Fig. 5–61. Pulsed Doppler recording in the descending aorta shows a normal velocity curve at 5 cm depth. At 6 cm increased velocity exceeding the limit for the pulsed mode is found. Recording with CW Doppler shows a maximal velocity of 3.6 m/s which gives a calculated peak pressure drop of 52 mm Hg across the coarctation.

traction. This pattern can be found when recording with pulsed Doppler from the right ventricle through the tricuspid orifice and into the right atrium (Figure 5.62). At 5 cm, recording is from the right ventricle since tricuspid flow velocity is recorded together with tricuspid valve opening. The partial valve closure in mid-diastole is also seen as well as reopening at atrial contraction, but closure at end-diastole is not recorded. At 6 cm the sampling volume is presumably at the area of the tricuspid orifice/right atrium, since tricuspid valve closure, but no longer valve opening, is clearly recorded. Diastolic flow velocity toward the transducer is still present, but now starts in late systole. It is recorded further back in the right atrium where tricuspid valve closure is no longer heard and flow velocity toward the transducer starts early in systole.

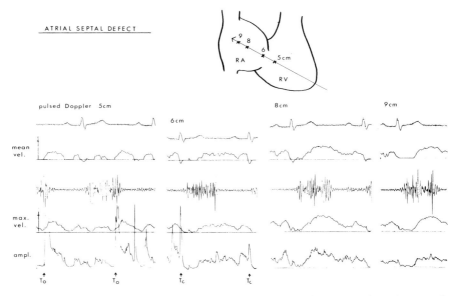

Fig. 5–62. In atrial septal defect, pulsed Doppler recording may show increased velocity of forward tricuspid flow. Recording behind the tricuspid valve in the right atrium shows that forward diastolic flow velocity is still recorded and here starts earlier, in mid-systole. Recording further back in the right atrium demonstrates that forward flow velocity starts early in systole, peaks at the second heart sound, and shows a second peak in late diastole following atrial contraction. To—tricuspid opening; Tc—tricuspid closure.

This velocity pattern has been found regularly in ASD. It was noted in 16 of 20 consecutive patients with ASD. The other four (60 to 75 years of age) all had significant tricuspid regurgitation changing the flow pattern in the right atrium in systole. In one patient, a velocity pattern of ASD, but with a higher velocity than usual, was recorded from the tricuspid valve up through the right atrium. The patient had an atrial septal aneurysm with a very small defect, and the higher velocity in the ASD flow was most likely due to a maintained pressure difference between the two atria. More striking, however, was the similarity between the movements of the septal aneurysm and the ASD flow pattern throughout the cardiac cycle (Figure 5.63). Maximal excursion of the aneurysm into the right atrium was in mid-to-late

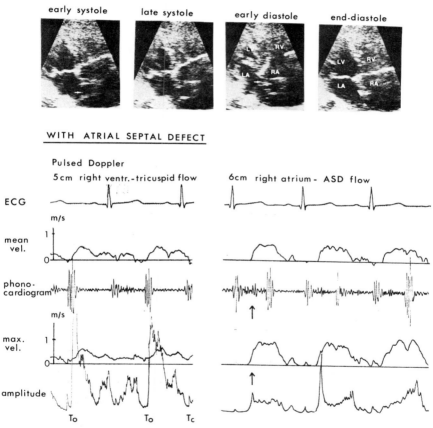

Fig. 5–63. The movements of an atrial septal aneurysm are seen to be similar to the flow pattern in ASD. It moves into the right atrium in early systole and with maximal excursion at end-systole. It starts to fold together in early to mid-diastole, and this is completed at end-diastole. Recording with Doppler showed that a small atrial septal defect was also present. Flow velocity into the right atrium was higher than usual suggesting a clear pressure difference between the two atria. It was preceded by a short click, presumably from the movement of the aneurysm into the right atrium. Lack of increase in flow velocity across the tricuspid valve also indicated that a left-to-right atrial shunt was insignificant.

systole, at the same time as velocity of ASD flow was highest and left-to-right atrial pressure difference presumably largest. At end-diastole both flow velocity and the excursion of the aneurysm were minimal, indicating equal pressures in the two atria.

The velocity pattern described may not be specific when recorded alone, since increased flow velocities in the right atrium may be recorded also with high cardiac output and with anomalous pulmonary venous drainage. The combination of Doppler and M-mode has been found helpful in the diagnosis of ASD,[61, 62] but combination with two-dimensional echocardiography would be expected to be much better.

With the increased flow through the right heart in ASD, velocity of flow across the right-sided valves increases. If one compares flow velocities recorded in the right and the left heart, the presence of left-to-right shunts at atrial level can be indicated and the ratio between velocities in the right and the left heart can be used to assess the magnitude of the shunt. In normal subjects, higher flow velocities are recorded through the mitral than through the tricuspid orifice, and higher in the aorta than in the pulmonary artery. The ratio between right- and left-sided velocities is usually 0.6 for both the atrioventricular valves and the great arteries. In ASD both tricuspid and pulmonary artery flow velocities are increased while mitral and aortic flow velocities in the lower normal range are usually recorded. Tricuspid flow velocity becomes as high or even higher than the mitral, and is more sustained throughout diastole. Pulmonary flow velocity is usually higher and may be two to three times as high as in the aorta.

Figure 5.64 is from a patient with a secundum atrial septal defect with a left-to-right shunt of 2.3:1. The pattern of ASD flow was recorded from the tricuspid orifice and 3 to 4 cm backward and upward in the right atrium. Flow velocity in the right ventricular outflow tract was as high as in the aorta and in the pulmonary artery more than twice as high. The increased tricuspid flow velocity makes the curve look more like a mitral flow curve while velocity of both mitral and aortic flow is lower than normal.

Figure 5.65 shows the ratio of right-to-left heart velocities in patients with ASD. It is compared to the ratio of flow through the pulmonary and the systemic circulation measured at catheterization. Following closure of the ASD, ratios between right and left heart velocities returned to the normal range. By measuring also the diameter of the aorta and the pulmonary artery, one might obtain a better estimate of shunt flow.

If mitral or tricuspid regurgitation is present in addition to ASD, this should be considered when comparing tricuspid and mitral flow velocities. As shown in Figure 5.65, velocity of tricuspid flow is relatively higher in relation to the size of the shunt in patients with tricuspid regurgitation.

In patients with left ventricular-right atrial shunts, velocity of both tricuspid and mitral flow is moderately increased and the ratio between them remains normal, whereas velocity of pulmonary flow is increased compared to aortic

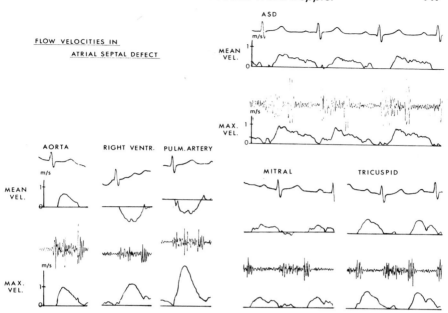

Fig. 5–64. Velocity of flow across the ASD and increased velocities across the tricuspid valve, in the right ventricle and in the pulmonary artery. Velocity of flow across both aortic and mitral valves is lower than usual.

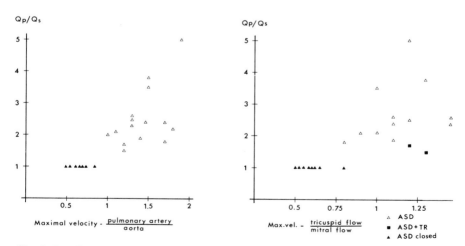

Fig. 5–65. Relation between tricuspid/mitral and pulmonary/aortic flow velocity and size of left-to-right shunt in 15 patients with ASD before operation and in 8 following surgical closure. Qp—pulmonary flow; Qs—systemic flow.

velocity. In patients with VSD and with more than small or moderate shunts, velocity of pulmonary flow is often higher than in the aorta, mitral flow velocity is increased, and tricuspid flow velocity is normal. One patient with an Eisenmenger syndrome due to a secundum atrial septal defect showed low velocities across all four valves and normal relation between the right and left heart. This compared well with catheterization data where cardiac output was low and a left-to-right shunt was no longer present.

5.7 OTHER CHANGES IN FLOW VELOCITY CURVES

A. Changes in Stroke Volume or Cardiac Output

In the absence of obstruction at the aortic valve area, velocity of flow in the ascending or descending aorta can give an indication of stroke volume or cardiac output. Changes in aortic flow velocity have been shown to correspond to changes in cardiac output.[63] As discussed in Section 2.1, stroke volume or cardiac output can be obtained if velocity of flow and the cross section of the ascending aorta can be measured, but the velocity profile then has to be flat where the measurements are made. Recording of aortic flow velocities is further discussed in Chapter 7. Problems in measuring cardiac output with this technique, therefore, include variations in velocities across the lumen in the ascending aorta where the velocity profile is assumed to be flat, changes in the cross-sectional area of the aorta during systole,[64] and the possible underestimation of velocity from a too-large angle to the velocity.

Several workers have reported good correlation between cardiac output or changes in stroke volume obtained by invasive methods and estimations made from velocities in the ascending aorta recorded noninvasively with Doppler.[65,65a,b] Comparisons between cardiac output from Doppler and from catheterization have also been reported using a combined Doppler and 2D-echo with the ultrasound beam from the left sternal border and the sample volume in the aortic root.[66]

Since aortic flow velocity can be rapidly obtained in many patients and changes in flow velocity correspond to changes in cardiac output, the circulation and circulatory changes in patients may be easily assessed. Figure 5.66 shows aortic flow velocity in a patient with a high output state, and the marked decrease in velocity with the decrease in cardiac output. When high cardiac output is present, high velocities can be recorded in both ventricles and great vessels in contrast to the shunts or regurgitations described earlier where increase in velocity is found across only one or two valves. In the patient in Figure 5.66 high velocities were recorded across the four valves and during systole in both ventricles, but were most marked in the ventricles and great arteries.

Buchtal, et al. have used CW Doppler recording of flow velocity in the aortic arch and have found this method to be useful for a quick assessment

Hyperkinetic heart syndrome

Noninvasive ultrasonic recording of flow

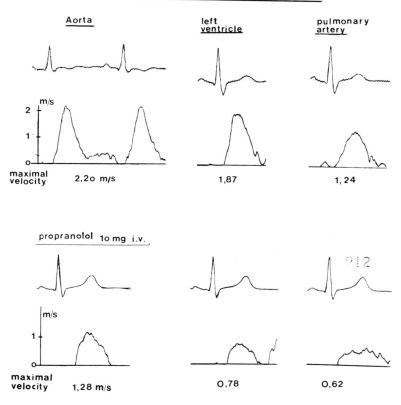

Cardiac output (Fick) 13,o l/min   (propranolol 4,o l/min)

Fig. 5–66. With high cardiac output, increased velocity of flow was recorded in the aorta, the left ventricle, and the pulmonary artery. There was no localized increase in velocity in the ventricle or at the aortic valve area, indicating that obstruction was not the cause of the increased velocity. Following administration of propranolol, cardiac output and velocity of flow were reduced.

of ill patients, as well as for the follow-up and judgment of therapy.[67] In the assessment they used peak velocity, the area under the velocity curve, and the shape of the curve.

Many patients with heart failure have low or low normal velocities in the aorta and across other valves. In three patients hospitalized with pronounced left and right heart failure, high velocities were recorded across all four heart valves. Figure 5.67 shows the velocities recorded in these three patients compared to velocities measured in other patients with heart failure. In all

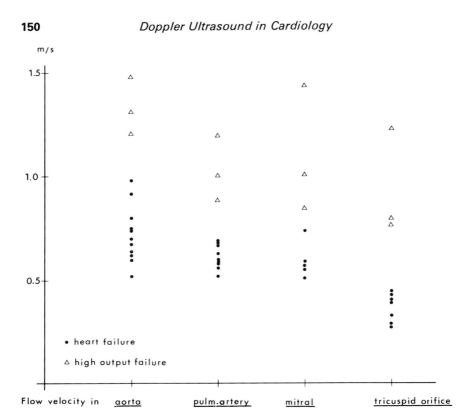

Fig. 5–67. Flow velocities recorded in three patients with high output failure, compared to flow velocities in other patients with heart failure.

three, thyrotoxicosis and high cardiac output were present. Since they had both mitral and tricuspid regurgitation which could partly explain the increased velocity across these valves, it was the high velocity in both the pulmonary artery and the aorta that indicated the increased cardiac output.

Instantaneous changes in aortic flow velocity are usually easy to detect. Changes with normal respiration are moderate and usually inapparent on examination. In Figure 5.68 increase in tricuspid flow velocity with inspiration is seen as normal, or even more clearly than usual, with normal respiration. In addition, this patient showed a clear variation in the Doppler signal from the ascending aorta with decrease at each inspiration. The change in the Doppler signal could not be explained as positional changes with respiration since a clear increase in preejection time and decrease in ejection time were seen together with the decrease in velocity, all probably due to reduced left ventricular filling during inspiration. Systolic blood pressure recorded simultaneously showed a decrease of 20 mm Hg with each inspiration. The patient had constrictive pericarditis. The recording of aortic

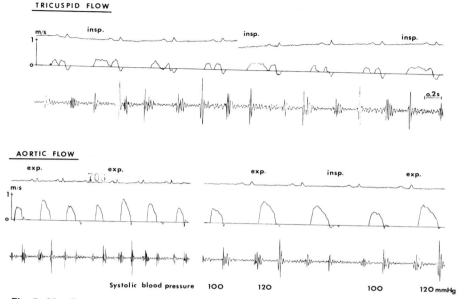

Fig. 5–68. Pulsed Doppler recording of tricuspid and aortic flow velocity in constrictive pericarditis. Tricuspid flow velocity increases with inspiration as normal, but in addition a clear decrease is noted in the audio signal and the recorded curve from the ascending aorta with each inspiration.

flow velocity demonstrated clearly that the decrease in velocity occurred immediately at each inspiration and not at one of the following beats as may occur in pulmonary diseases.

Figure 5.69 is from another patient in whom a clear variation in the Doppler signal from the ascending aorta was easily heard from beat to beat. In this patient, reduced velocity was noted in every second beat except for premature beats, and there was no relation to respiration. The patient was in severe heart failure and an alternating pulse was palpable. Changes in systolic time intervals were seen together with changes in velocity. Similar velocity recordings in pulsus alternans have been reported from invasive measurements.[68]

B. Changes in Aortic and Pulmonary Flow Velocity Curves

The shape of the aortic flow velocity curve is determined by cardiac function as well as by the capacitance and resistance of the systemic arteries. Changes in the aortic flow velocity curves are therefore seen in a variety of heart lesions. Changes in hypertrophic cardiomyopathy,[47] in mitral regurgitation,[36] and in shock[67] have been described. In left heart failure, a lower velocity is often combined with a slower increase in velocity,

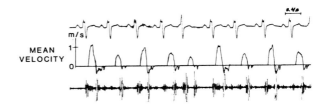

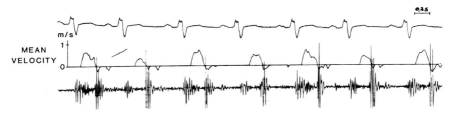

Fig. 5–69. Pulsed Doppler recording of flow velocity in the ascending aorta in a patient with severe heart failure and pulsus alternans. The difference in the Doppler signal for every second beat was clearly heard.

a more rounded curve form, and peak velocity later in systole. Similar aortic flow velocity curves can also be seen in patients with normal left ventricular function. They have been found in conditions with decreased left ventricular filling (severe mitral stenosis, atrial septal defect, and primary pulmonary hypertension) and in conditions with a dilated ascending aorta, such as Marfan's syndrome or Fallot's tetralogy. Figure 5.70 shows examples of changed aortic flow velocity curves compared to normal. Figure 5.71 shows both decrease in velocity and changed curve form in ventricular premature

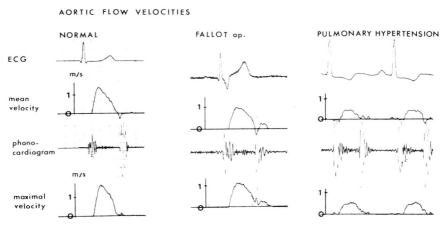

Fig. 5–70. Changes in aortic flow velocity curves. The curve to the right is from a patient with severe primary pulmonary hypertension.

beats compared to sinus beats. The recording is from a healthy 13-year-old child. Elzinga and Westerhof, in an experimental study, have recorded the changes in pressure and flow in the ascending aorta resulting from changes in capacitance and resistance.[69] Mean and peak velocity decreased with both decreased capacitance and increased resistance. A change in the form of the flow velocity curve was also seen with both decreased capacitance and increased resistance. During the Valsalva maneuver, significant changes in aortic flow velocity and pressure curves in man have been shown to be due to changes in wave reflections in the arterial tree.[70] Attempts to assess left ventricular function from aortic flow velocity curves have been described using catheter-tip velocity transducers.[71, 72] A more extensive analysis of the aortic flow velocity curve in experimental and various clinical conditions and the result of changes in these might yield useful information. The aortic flow velocity curve could become an important parameter in assessment of both left ventricular function and the arterial system.

AORTIC FLOW VELOCITY

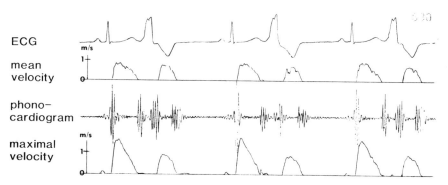

Fig. 5–71. Change in configuration of aortic flow velocity curve from sinus beats to ventricular premature beats in a healthy subject.

Changes in *pulmonary* flow velocity curves have been less adequately described. When flow velocity curves from the pulmonary artery were recorded with Doppler, it was noticed that patients with pulmonary hypertension and significantly raised pulmonary vascular resistance did not exhibit the usual rounded curve with peak velocity nearly at mid-systole. Figure 5.72 shows flow velocity curves from the aorta and the pulmonary artery in a normal subject and one patient with pulmonary hypertension. The flow velocity curve from the pulmonary artery in pulmonary hypertension shows an early peak followed by a rapid decrease in velocity and early cessation of flow. It resembles an aortic flow velocity curve. The pulmonary vascular resistance in this patient was higher than the systemic. The aortic flow velocity curve is more rounded with a later peak velocity than in the normal subject. The late pulmonary valve opening coincides with an early systolic

NORMAL SUBJECT

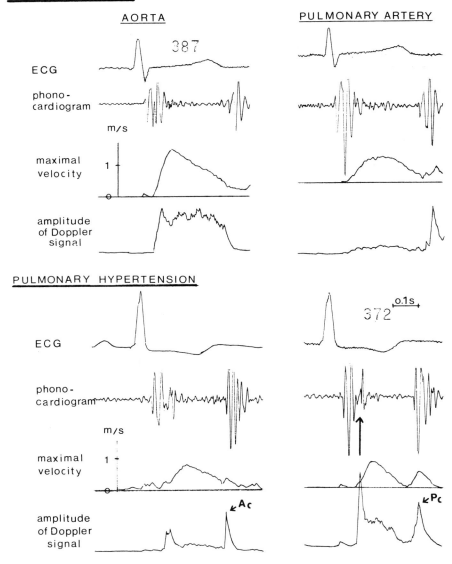

Fig. 5–72. A normal maximal velocity curve from the pulmonary artery has a more rounded form with lower and later peak velocity than in the aorta. In pulmonary hypertension with increased pulmonary vascular resistance, the maximal velocity curve from the pulmonary artery shows an earlier peak, and earlier and more rapid decrease in velocity. The curve resembles an aortic flow velocity curve. Aortic flow velocity is also changed with lower and later peak velocity than normal. P_c—pulmonary valve closure; A_c—aortic valve closure.

click (arrow). Similar velocity patterns in the pulmonary artery have been recorded in many patients with pulmonary hypertension and increased resistance. In some, the velocity curves have even resembled those presented by Elzinga and Westerhof from the aorta following experimentally decreased capacitance and increased resistance,[69] and it seems reasonable to assume that the observed changes are caused by changes in the pulmonary vascular bed. Similar velocity curves have not been observed in the pulmonary artery in normal individuals or in patients with increased pulmonary artery pressure without increased resistance.[22] A similar flow pattern in the pulmonary artery in pulmonary hypertension has been shown using contrast echocardiography[69a] and by recording pulmonary flow velocity invasively[69b] and noninvasively with pulsed Doppler.[69c]

C.   Changes in Atrioventricular Flow Velocity Curves

The changes seen in the mitral flow velocity curves in hypertrophic cardiomyopathy have been described in Section 5.4. Figure 5.73 illustrates these changes with the increased velocity following atrial contraction and the slower decrease in early diastolic velocity compared to normal. This velocity pattern is regularly found in patients with significant left ventricular hypertrophy and a small or nondilated ventricular cavity, as in hypertrophic cardiomyopathy and aortic valve stenosis. It is not seen in patients with hypertrophy and dilated left ventricles, as in aortic regurgitation.

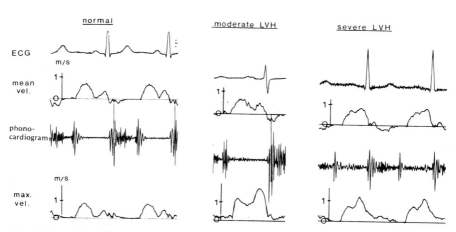

Fig. 5–73.   **Mitral flow velocity in a normal subject, in one patient with moderate left ventricular hypertrophy (LVH), and in one with severe LVH. The increase in velocity following atrial contraction is more pronounced in LVH. In severe LVH both mean and maximal velocities are higher than earlier in diastole.**

In tricuspid flow, the velocity early in diastole and at atrial contraction may be of similar height, especially during inspiration when the latter may even be a little higher. In moderate right ventricular hypertrophy, this can be seen in both respiratory phases. The pattern resembles that found in normal neonates as described in Chapter 4. With pronounced right ventricular hypertrophy, a pattern as seen to the right in Figure 5.74 may be found.

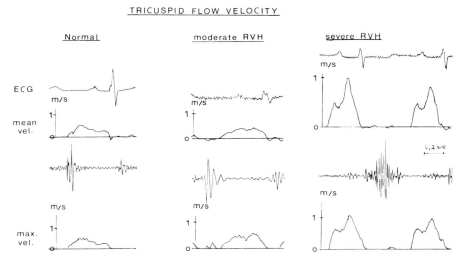

Fig. 5–74. In right ventricular hypertrophy (RVH), increase in tricuspid flow velocity following atrial contraction is more pronounced than in normal individuals. The curve to the right is from an adult with severe pulmonary valve stenosis.

The difference between normal mitral and tricuspid flow velocity curves may be due to left atrial pressure being higher than the right, with a higher pressure drop present in early diastole across the mitral than the tricuspid valve. Flow velocity curves recorded from patients after operation with Mustard's procedure for transposition of the great arteries seem to confirm this. In Figure 5.75, the flow velocity curve through the tricuspid valve (pulmonary venous return) resembles a normal mitral flow velocity curve, whereas the curve recorded at the mitral valve (systemic venous return) resembles a normal tricuspid flow velocity curve, with respiratory variation clearly heard in the audio signal.

The relation between mitral and tricuspid flow velocity curves may also be changed by increases in flow across one of the valves as described with valvular regurgitations or shunts. Figure 5.76 shows decrease in mitral flow velocity with reduced cardiac output, while tricuspid flow velocity is not reduced because of tricuspid regurgitation, a short diastole due to pulmonary hypertension, and an increased a-wave due to pronounced right ventricular hypertrophy.

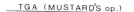

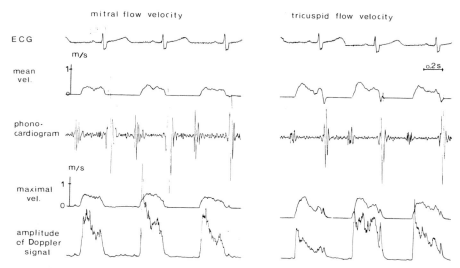

Fig. 5–75. Following Mustard's operation for transposition of the great arteries (TGA), the normal patterns of mitral and tricuspid flow velocities are exchanged. The mitral flow velocity now shows increase during inspiration, and the velocity curve looks like a normal tricuspid flow velocity curve, while the tricuspid looks like a normal mitral flow velocity curve.

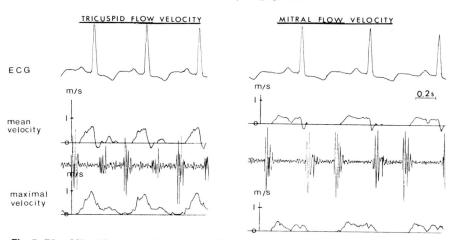

Fig. 5–76. Mitral flow velocity is reduced in this patient with pulmonary hypertension and a very low cardiac output. Tricuspid flow velocity is not reduced owing to tricuspid regurgitation, increased velocity following atrial contraction (severe right ventricular hypertrophy), and the short filling period (late opening of tricuspid valve due to the high pulmonary artery pressure).

The effects of atrial arrhythmias on atrioventricular velocity curves are easily seen. Figure 5.77 shows the increase in velocity in tricuspid flow following each atrial contraction in atrial flutter and the change in a mitral flow velocity curve with change from nodal to sinus rhythm. Figure 5.78 illustrates the short diastolic filling period during ventricular tachycardia in a patient with mitral stenosis.

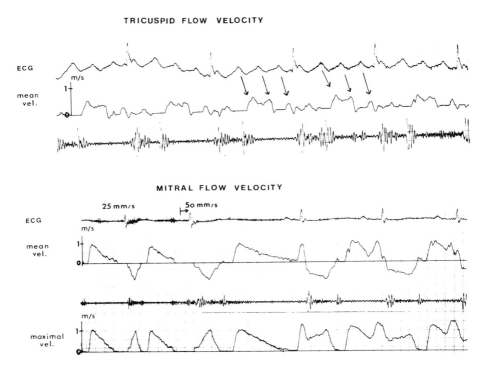

Fig. 5–77. Effect of atrial arrhythmias on atrioventricular flow velocity curves. With atrial flutter the effect of repeated contractions is seen (upper curve) and in nodal rhythm the second peak is missing (lower curve).

5.8   VALVE MOVEMENTS

Since valve movements are usually clearly shown in the amplitude curve, this can be used for timing of intracardiac events. During recording at the valve areas, start of the valve opening and end of the closing movement can usually be clearly defined for both the left- and right-sided valves in both children and adults. This makes it possible to obtain right heart systolic time intervals easily in most patients. The right ventricular isovolumetric relaxation time has been used to estimate systolic pulmonary artery pressure by the Burstin method,[29, 30] and good correlation with pressures recorded at cathe-

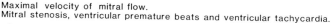

Maximal velocity of mitral flow.
Mitral stenosis, ventricular premature beats and ventricular tachycardia.

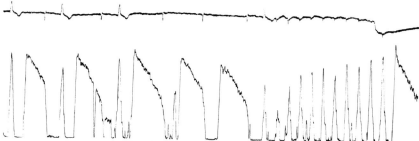

Fig. 5–78. Effect of tachycardia on the diastolic filling time in a patient with mitral stenosis.

terization was obtained in both children and adults. The method assumes that right atrial pressure is normal; therefore, in patients with significantly increased right atrial pressure, underestimation of pulmonary artery pressure may occur. In patients with right heart failure, good correlation with pressure recording has still been obtained. This might be due to a slower right ventricular relaxation rate that might balance the effect of a significantly raised right atrial pressure on the estimated pulmonary artery pressure. In patients with mild to moderate tricuspid regurgitation, estimated pressures have been close to recorded pressures, but in patients with more than moderate tricuspid regurgitation, pulmonary artery pressure has been significantly underestimated in most. Even when an increased right atrial pressure was added, it was still underestimated in some, indicating that changes in right ventricular relaxation rate might also be present. In patients with significant tricuspid regurgitation, however, calculation of a right ventricular-right atrial pressure difference in systole from maximal velocity in the tricuspid regurgitation usually shows whether right ventricular pressure is raised.

Even in aortic valve stenosis with calcified valves, the opening and closing movements can in almost all cases be recorded and left ventricular ejection time assessed. Good correlation has been shown between systolic time intervals obtained from Doppler, from carotid artery curves, and from aortic and pulmonary valve movements recorded with M-mode.[73]

In patients with prosthetic (disc) valves, however, problems may occur in timing of the other valve movements, since the strong reflections from the disc movements can usually be recorded at positions quite a distance from the prosthesis.

The combined recording of valve movements with the phonocardiogram is useful, as has been shown with the combined use of M-mode and phonocardiogram. The simultaneous flow velocity measurements give added information. Figure 5.79 is from a young patient admitted with heart failure of unknown etiology. No diastolic murmur was heard or recorded, and the

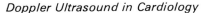

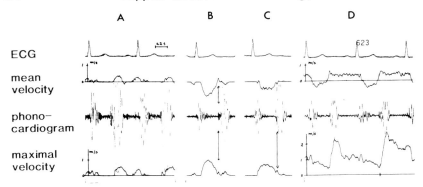

Fig. 5–79.   A, Tricuspid flow velocity. B and C, Flow velocity at aortic and pulmonary valve areas with valve closures. D, Aortic regurgitation.

second heart sound was thought to be both loud and prolonged. Tricuspid flow started earlier than the second sound. Pulmonary and aortic valve closures were also earlier with almost no sound. This was overshadowed by a very prominent third heart sound found to coincide with peak velocity of a large aortic regurgitation.

"Abnormal" valve motions, such as valve flutter, are easily detected. The diastolic flutter of the mitral valve in aortic regurgitation and in conditions with increased mitral flow and the diastolic and systolic flutter in flail mitral leaflet have been described. Pronounced diastolic flutter of the mitral valve was also found in one patient with left atrial myxoma, which has also been described with M-mode.[11c] Diastolic flutter of the tricuspid valve has been noted in pulmonary regurgitation, in the early filling period in ASD with large left-to-right shunts, and in patients with mild tricuspid stenosis following de Vega's annuloplasty. Systolic flutter of the tricuspid valve has been found in ventricular septal defects as well as in left ventricular-right atrial shunts.

Both aortic and pulmonary valve flutter have been recorded in many young, normal subjects. Pulmonary valve flutter has been found regularly in pulmonary hypertension, and aortic valve flutter occurs regularly in sub-valvular aortic stenosis, but also in some patients with aortic valve stenosis. A pronounced flutter of the aortic valve has been noted in some subjects with a harsh loud systolic murmur where no other reason for the murmur could be found. Figure 5.80, which is from such a patient, shows that the frequency of the valve flutter is equal to that of the murmur on the phonocardiogram. A similar relation can be seen in Figure 5.48 between the frequency of the flutter of the disc valve and that of the systolic murmur. The subject in Figure 5.80 showed no sign of subvalvular obstruction or increased cardiac output. Both systolic and diastolic flutter of the pulmonary valve are found in some patients with patent ductus arteriosus.

SYSTOLIC FLUTTER OF AORTIC VALVE

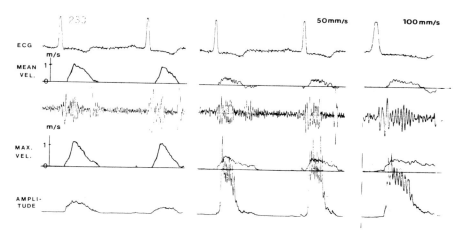

Fig. 5–80.   Systolic murmur in patient with no signs of heart disease. The frequency of the murmur in the phonocardiogram is the same as the frequency of the valve flutter (amplitude curve).

5.9   USEFULNESS, PROBLEMS, AND LIMITATIONS

A.   Usefulness

In mitral stenosis where the method was first applied, the degree of obstruction can usually be clearly shown today with 2D echocardiography. The use of both methods provides added information since data on both pressure drop and valve area give an indication of the flow across the valve. In aortic valve stenosis, a good estimation of the pressure drop is obtained in young patients in whom the valve lesion is usually fairly easy to detect and assess with 2D echocardiography. In such cases, however, the Doppler seems easier to use and information on the pressure drop in addition to the valve area is useful. In older patients, the jet can be more difficult to find and the pressure drop underestimated. From the Doppler signal, it is usually evident whether a reasonable estimate of the maximal velocity is obtained or not and, combined with the shape of the velocity curve, the degree of obstruction can be assessed in about 80%. Again the use of both Doppler and echocardiography helps to assess the lesion correctly in more patients. Because of the different positions and angles used, it may be easy to record the valve area clearly in a patient in whom the jet is difficult to record and vice versa. An area where Doppler contributes more to the clinical and echocardiographic evaluation is in the diagnosis and assessment of valve regurgitations. We have been surprised at the number of valve regurgitations diagnosed with Doppler where this was not suspected from the clinical examination, since either no murmur was heard or recorded, a very weak murmur was considered to be without significance, or the patient had a murmur from another lesion. Examples of the first have been aortic regurgitation in bacterial endocarditis and both tricuspid and mitral regurgitation, which have been shown in patients with no audible or insignificant murmurs. The presence of mitral regurgitation in addition to aortic valve stenosis is easily shown, as well as the presence of both mitral and tricuspid regurgitation in mitral stenosis or secondary to left heart failure.

Another area where Doppler adds significantly to the clinical and echocardiographic evaluation is in patients with prosthetic valves, since echocardiography is less helpful in the evaluation of prostheses than of ordinary valves. The possibility of a noninvasive diagnosis of pulmonary hypertension contributes to the clinical evaluation and helps in a correct timing of eventual catheter studies and surgery.

In children, the Doppler technique is useful by excluding abnormalities in evaluation of systolic murmurs. In congenital heart disease, it complements echocardiography, the techniques often being equally useful. Echocardiography is more useful in some patients and Doppler in some. The Doppler technique seems especially helpful in diagnosis or exclusion of associated lesions, and in evaluation following surgery, whether residual murmurs are present or not.

Another field where the technique could become useful is in the diagnosis and assessment of patent ductus arteriosus in premature infants. Further evaluation of the technique is necessary in these patients.

There has been great interest in the possibility of measuring cardiac output. This still presents problems, but relative changes are fairly easy to assess. Similarly, the relation between flow velocities in the right and left sides of the heart can be helpful to show differences in flow and thereby to assess the degree of left-to-right shunts.

B. Problems and Limitations

To record velocity of blood flow, the necessity of obtaining a small angle to the velocity is the main problem. As described, the audio signal can be a useful guide for obtaining a small angle, but it is also the best indicator of the presence of a too-large angle to a velocity. The older patients with aortic valve stenosis present the greatest problems, since the jet in these patients may have very different directions, and it may not be possible to obtain a small angle. The combined use of 2D echocardiography and Doppler should help to obtain a good direction, but since a longitudinal plane through a ventricle or an artery still may be at an angle to the velocity, the audio signal should still be used to find the best direction. In patients with complex anatomy, localization from the Doppler signal alone may present problems, and the combined use of 2D echocardiography and Doppler may be necessary or preferable. Using a Doppler alone may still be helpful by showing flow in two different great arteries and through two different A-V valves.

The maximum Doppler shift is a main parameter for evaluation of many lesions. For optimal results with the estimator described in Section 3.5A, one has to pay attention to the gain setting. With good Doppler signals, the gain setting does not present problems as there is a wide range from a gain setting where the Doppler signal is adequately recorded to a too-high gain setting where noise interferes (Figure 3.16). If Doppler signals are weak or if only a few of the highest frequencies are present in the signal, a higher gain setting may be necessary and may come to the level where noise disturbs the recording. There are situations where weak high-frequency signals are clearly heard but cannot be recorded since the maximal frequency estimator may follow the noise and thereby indicate a falsely high velocity. Spectral analysis may sometimes help in recording such signals, but it is in most cases equally difficult to get a clear outline of the spectrum.

Fortunately, weak Doppler signals or those with only few high frequencies are mainly found at larger depths and in regurgitant jets where the amount of regurgitation is small and therefore less important. However, it can also be a problem in some of the older patients with aortic valve stenosis where only part of the aortic jet may be reached with the ultrasound beam and the lower frequencies therefore dominate the Doppler signal.

An example is shown in Figure 5.81. By a gradual increase in gain from the first to the third beat, a higher maximal velocity is recorded, but in the next three beats the gain setting becomes too high with artifacts in the velocity curve due to noise. It is, therefore, important to listen to the audio signal while recording. The presence of artifacts may also be seen from the recorded curves. With an adequate Doppler signal, a smooth rounded curve should be obtained in both obstructions and regurgitations. With a less clear signal, the highest velocities may not be recorded and the curve may have a cut-off appearance as with a pulsed Doppler recording, but mean and maximal velocities and the amplitude curve show a similar time course. When artifacts are present, the maximal velocity curve increases or continues longer than it should, such as past A2 in aortic stenosis or beyond the time where the amplitude decreases, as shown in Figure 5.81. This is clearly seen when comparing maximal velocity and amplitude in Figures 5.25 and 5.81. In contrast to the artifacts seen in Figure 5.81, both maximal velocity and amplitude in Figure 5.25 continue to a delayed P_2 both when high velocities are recorded and when they are partly lost.

If high frequencies are heard in the audio signal but are difficult to record without artifacts in the maximal velocity curve, a position with more higher frequencies and fewer lower frequencies should be attempted. This is especially important if the low frequencies are of high intensity as in VSD or with fluttering valves. In such cases, the gain may have to be turned so low that

AORTIC STENOSIS - CW DOPPLER

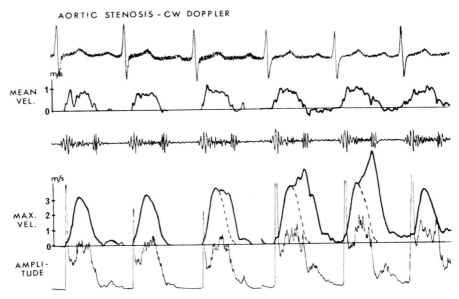

Fig. 5–81. Artifacts in the maximal velocity curve (third to fifth beat) seen when increasing gain in order to record the maximal frequencies present in the Doppler signal. In the third beat, a slightly higher maximal velocity is recorded, but the estimator also reacts to noise, and artifacts are seen in this and the two following beats. Loss of the normally rounded curve form seen in beats 1, 2 and 6 with increased gain, and continuation of the maximal velocity curve beyond the amplitude and the mean velocity curve indicate the presence of artifacts. The stippled line indicates what the course of the velocity curve should have been.

no high velocities can be recorded. Figure 5.82 is from a patient with a ventricular septal defect where "gain" is gradually increased from a very low level. The maximal velocity recorded increases in the first three beats, and a sharp decrease in maximal velocity is seen at the beginning of the second heart sound and simultaneous with decrease in the amplitude. In the two last beats with the artifacts, the maximal velocity curve continues longer and no longer follows the amplitude curve.

Both with weak and with too strong signals where the recording is disturbed by noise or by low frequencies of high intensity, the filter with highest cut-off frequency should be used. With fewer low frequencies in the signal, higher frequencies may be more easily recorded. This filter should not be used while searching for a good signal, since the lower frequencies are masked and this may cause a false impression of a good signal. When low velocities are present as in the reverse flow velocity in the aorta in aortic regurgitation, the filter with the lowest cut-off frequency should be used; otherwise, these may not be recorded.

VSD - CW DOPPLER - increase in "gain" ⟶

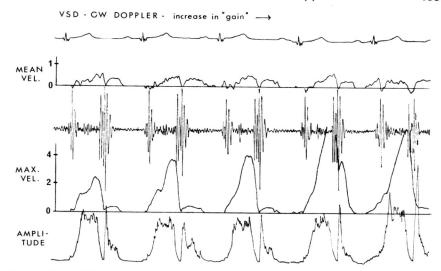

Fig. 5–82. In VSD a strong signal often produces artifacts in the maximal velocity curve unless the "gain" is set very low. High frequencies present in the Doppler signal may then fail to be recorded as in the first beat. With a slight increase in gain, higher velocities are recorded in the third beat, while in the next two beats artifacts occur. Decrease in maximal velocity is seen to occur simultaneously with decrease in amplitude, but continues longer in the presence of artifacts in the last two beats.

Since the pulsed mode has a better signal-to-noise ratio than the continuous mode, weak signals may be easier to record with the pulsed mode. Since most of the information is from the maximal velocities, however, the pulsed mode is of less help. With possibilities to record higher velocities in the pulsed mode as discussed in Chapter 6, the recording of weak high-frequency Doppler signals may be improved. The limitations discussed in Section 5.5, when two different high-velocity jets are present, can also be overcome by capabilities to record higher velocities in the pulsed mode.

Some of the problems and limitations with the present technique may be partly overcome by the combined use of 2D echocardiography and Doppler, but for optimal Doppler recordings one should still be able to use the technique separately. CW Doppler would still be useful in searching for abnormal flow signals and high-velocity jets and in recording the highest velocities.

REFERENCES

1. Hatle L., Brubakk A., Tromsdal A., Angelsen B.: Noninvasive assessment of pressure drop in mitral stenosis by Doppler ultrasound. Br. Heart J. 1978; 40: 131-140.
2. Hatle L., Angelsen B., Tromsdal A.: Noninvasive assessment of atrioventricular pressure half-time by Doppler ultrasound. Circulation 1979; 60: 1096-1104.

3. Holen J., Aaslid R., Landmark K., Simonsen S.: Determination of pressure gradient in mitral stenosis with a noninvasive ultrasound Doppler technique. Acta Med. Scand. 1976; 199: 455-460.
4. Holen J., Simonsen S.: Determination of pressure gradient in mitral stenosis with Doppler echocardiography. Br. Heart J. 1979; 41: 529-535.
5. Hatle L., Angelsen B.A., Tromsdal A.: Noninvasive assessment of aortic stenosis by Doppler ultrasound. Br. Heart J. 1980; 43: 284-292.
6. Hatle L.: Noninvasive assessment and differentiation of left ventricular outflow obstruction by Doppler ultrasound. Circulation 1981; 64: 381-387.
7. Holen J., Aaslid R., Landmark K., Simonsen S., Østrem T.: Determination of effective orifice area in mitral stenosis from noninvasive ultrasound Doppler data and mitral flow rate. Acta Med. Scand. 1977; 201: 83-88.
8. Murgo J.P., Altobelli S.A., Dorethy J.F., Logsdon J.R., McGranahan G.H.: Normal ventricular ejection dynamics in man during rest and exercise. In: Physiologic Principles of Heart Sounds and Murmurs. Edited by Leon S.F., Shaver J.A. Dallas, American Heart Association 1975; 92-101.
9. Løken M.: Parameter estimation in nonlinear heart model. Thesis (in Norwegian). Division of Eng. Cybernetics, The Norwegian Institute of Technology, Trondheim, Norway, 1979.
10. Kalmanson D.,Veyrat C., Bouchareine F., Degroote A.: Noninvasive recording of mitral valve flow velocity patterns using pulsed Doppler echocardiography. Br. Heart J. 1977; 39: 517-528.
11. Thuillez C., Théroux P., Bourassa M.G., Blanchard D., et al.: Pulsed Doppler echocardiographic study of mitral stenosis. Circulation 1980; 61: 381-387.
11a. Boughner D.R., Persaüd J.A.: Transcutaneous continuous wave Doppler ultrasound in the diagnosis of left atrial myxoma. Chest 1981; 79: 322-326.
11b. Niederle P., Stepánek Z., Grospie A., Ressl J., Firt P., Beránek I., Dubovska M.: Character of mitral valve flow in left atrial tumor. Eur. J. Cardiol. 1981; 12: 357-365.
11c. Ciraulo D.: Mitral valve fluttering. An echocardiographic feature of left atrial myxoma. Chest 1979; 76: 95-96.
11d. Hatle, L.: Noninvasive assessment of aortic stenosis in adults with Doppler ultrasound. In press, 1982.
12. Young J.B., Quinones M.A., Waggoner A.D., Miller R.R.: Diagnosis and quantification of aortic stenosis with pulsed Doppler echocardiography. Am. J. Cardiol. 1980; 45: 987-994.
13. Veyrat C., Cholot N., Abitbol G., Kalmanson D.: Validity of echo-pulsed Doppler velocimetry for assessing the diagnosis and severity of aortic valve disease and prosthetic valve function. In: Echocardiology. Edited by Lancée C.T. Hague, Martinus Nijhoff, 1979; 261-266.
14. Veyrat C., Cholot N., Abitbol G., Kalmanson D.: Noninvasive diagnosis and assessment of aortic valve disease and evaluation of aortic prosthesis function using echo pulsed Doppler velocimetry. Br. Heart J. 1980; 43: 393-413.
14a. Kawabori I., Stevenson J.G., Dooley T.K., Phillips D.J., Sylvester C.M., Guntheroth W.G.: The significance of carotid bruits in children: transmitted murmur of vascular origin, studies by pulsed Doppler ultrasound. Am. Heart J. 1979; 98: 160-167.
14b. Kawabori I., Stevenson J.G., Dooley T.K., Guntheroth W.G.: Evaluation of ejection murmurs by pulsed Doppler echocardiography. Br. Heart J. 1980; 43: 623-628.
14c. Goldberg S.J., Areias J., Feldman L., Sahn D.J., Allen H. D.: Lesions that cause aortic flow disturbance. Circulation 1979; 60: 1539-1547.
14d. Cumming G.R.: Second heart sound after pulmonary arterial banding procedure. Br. Heart J. 1976; 38: 497-503.
14e. Finnegan P., Ihenacho H.N.C., Singh S.P., Abrams L.D.: Haemodynamic studies at rest and during exercise in pulmonary stenosis after surgery. Br. Heart J. 1974; 36: 913-918.
14f. Goldberg S.J., Areias J.C., Spitaels S.E.C., de Villeneuve V.H.: Echo Doppler detection of pulmonary stenosis by time interval histogram analysis. J. Clin. Ultrasound 1979; 7: 183-189.
14g. Areias J.C., Goldberg S.J., Spitaels S.E.C., de Villeneuve V.H.: An evaluation of range-gated pulsed Doppler echocardiography for detecting pulmonary outflow tract obstruction in d-transposition of the great vessels. Am. Heart J. 1978; 96: 467-474.
15. Haerten K., Seipel L., Loogen F., Herzer J.: Haemodynamic studies after De Vega's tricuspid annuloplasty. Circulation 1978; 58: 28-33.

16. Boughner D.R.: Assessment of aortic insufficiency by transcutaneous Doppler ultrasound. Circulation 1975; 52: 874-879.

16a. Ward J.M., Baker D.W., Rubenstein S.A., Johnson S.L.: Detection of aortic insufficiency by pulsed Doppler echocardiography. J. Clin. Ultrasound 1977; 5: 5-10.

16b. Brubakk A.O., Angelsen B.A.J., Hatle L.: Diagnosis of valvular heart disease using transcutaneous Doppler ultrasound. Cardiovasc. Res. 1977; 11: 461-469.

16c. Gross B.W., Franklin D.W., Pearlman S.: Improved non-invasive detection of aortic insufficiency in patients with mitral stenosis using pulsed Doppler echocardiography. Circulation 1981; 64 (Suppl. IV): 256 (Abstract).

17. Sequeira R.F., Watt J.: Assessment of aortic regurgitation by transcutaneous aortovelography. Br. Heart J. 1977; 39: 929.

18. Jenni R., Hübscher W., Casty M., Anliker M., Krayenbuehl H.P.: Quantitation of aortic regurgitation by a percutaneous 128-channel digital ultrasound Doppler instrument. *In:* Echocardiology. Edited by Lancée C.T. Hague, Martinus Nijhoff, 1979; 241-243.

19. Quinones M.A., Young J.B., Waggoner A.D., Ostojic M.C., Ribeiro L.G.T., Miller R.R.: Assessment of pulsed Doppler echocardiography in detection and quantification of aortic and mitral regurgitation. Br. Heart J. 1980; 44: 612-620.

19a. Hatteland K., Semb B.: Assessment of aortic regurgitation by means of pulsed Doppler ultrasound. Ultrasound Med. Biol. In press, 1982.

20. Tunstall Pedoe D.S.: Blood velocity measurements in aortic regurgitation using heated thin film and ultrasonic techniques. Br. Heart J. 1971; 33:611.

21. Garcia-Dorado Garcia A.D., Lopez Bescos L., Almazan Ceballos A., Alvarez Diaz R.: Velocimetria Doppler transcutanea de la arteria subclavia en el estudio de la valvulopathia aortica. Revista Española de Cardiologia 1980; 33: 249-257.

21a. Nimura Y., Matsuo H., Hayashi T., Kitabatake A., Mochizuki S., Sakakibara H., Kato K., Abe H.: Studies on arterial flow patterns—instantaneous velocity spectrums and their phasic changes—with directional ultrasonic Doppler technique. Br. Heart J. 1974; 36: 899-907.

21b. Risöe C., Wille S.Ø.: Blood velocity in human arteries measured by a bidirectional ultrasonic Doppler flowmeter. Acta Physiol. Scand. 1978; 103: 370-378.

22. Hatle L.: Changes in pulmonary flow velocity curves in pulmonary hypertension. To be published.

23. Benchimol A., Stegall H.F., Gartlan J.L.: New method to measure phasic coronary blood velocity in man. Am. Heart J. 1971; 81: 93-101.

24. Skjærpe T., Hatle L.: Diagnosis and assessment of tricuspid regurgitation with Doppler ultrasound. *In:* Echocardiology. Edited by Rijsterborgh H. Hague, Martinus Nijhoff, 1981; 299-304.

25. Benchimol A., Harris C.L., Desser K.B.: Noninvasive diagnosis of tricuspid insufficiency utilizing the external Doppler flowmeter probe. Am. J. Cardiol. 1973; 32: 868-873.

26. Baker D.W., Rubenstein S.A., Lorch G.S.: Pulsed Doppler echocardiography: Principles and applications. Am. J. Med. 1977; 63: 69-80.

27. Fantini F., Magherini A.: Detection of tricuspid regurgitation with pulsed Doppler echocardiography. *In:* Echocardiology. Edited by Lancée C.T. Hague, Martinus Nijhoff, 1979; 233-235.

27a. Stevenson G., Kawabori I., Guntheroth W.: Validation of Doppler diagnosis of tricuspid regurgitation. Circulation 1981; 64 (Suppl. IV): 255 (Abstract).

27b. Lieppe W., Behar V.S., Scallion R., Kisslo J.A.: Detection of tricuspid regurgitation with two-dimensional echocardiography and peripheral vein injection. Circulation 1978; 57: 128.

27c. Meltzer R.S., van Hoogenhuyze D., Serruys P.W., Haalebos M.M.P., Hugenholtz P.G., Roelandt J.: Diagnosis of tricuspid regurgitation by contrast echocardiography. Circulation 1981; 63: 1093-1099.

27d. Skjærpe T.: Diagnosis of tricuspid regurgitation, sensitivity of Doppler compared to contrast echocardiography. To be published.

27e. Goldberg S.J., Valdes-Cruz L.M., Feldman L., Sahn D.J., Allen H.D.: Range-gated Doppler ultrasound detection of contrast echocardiographic microbubbles for cardiac and great vessel blood flow patterns. Am. Heart J. 1981; 101: 793-796.

27f. Sakakibara H., Miyatake K., Okamoto M., Kinoshita N., Nimura Y.: Noninvasive assessment of severity of tricuspid regurgitation with a combined use of the ultrasonic pulsed

Doppler technique and two-dimensional echocardiography. Circulation 1980; 62 (Suppl. III): 250 (Abstract).

27g. Stevenson J.G., Kawabori I., Brandestini M.A.: A twenty-month experience comparing conventional pulsed Doppler echocardiography and color-coded digital multigate Doppler for detection of atrioventricular valve regurgitation and its severity. *In:* Echocardiology. Edited by Rijsterborgh H. Hague, Martinus Nijhoff, 1981; 399-407.

27h. Blanchard D., Diebold B., Guermonprez J.L., Peronneau P., Forman J., Maurice P.: Noninvasive quantification of tricuspid regurgitation by Doppler echocardiography. Circulation 1981; 64 (Suppl. IV): 256 (Abstract).

28. Braunwald E., Awe W.C.: The syndrome of severe mitral regurgitation with normal left atrial pressure. Circulation 1963; 27: 29-35.

29. Burstin L.: Determination of pressure in the pulmonary artery by external graphic recordings. Br. Heart J. 1967; 29: 396-404.

30. Hatle L., Angelsen B.A.J., Tromsdal A.: Noninvasive estimation of pulmonary artery systolic pressure with Doppler ultrasound. Br. Heart J. 1981; 45: 157-165.

31. Johnson S.L., Baker D.W., Lute R.A., Murray J.A.: Detection of mitral regurgitation by Doppler echocardiography (Abstract). Am. J. Cardiol. 1974; 33: 146.

32. Stevenson J.G., Kawabori I., Guntheroth W.G.: Differentiation of ventricular septal defects from mitral regurgitation by pulsed Doppler echocardiography. Circulation 1977; 56: 14-18.

33. Abbasi A.S., Allen M.W., De Christofaro D., Ungar J.: Detection and estimation of the degree of mitral regurgitation by range-gated pulsed Doppler echocardiography. Circulation 1980; 61: 143-147.

33a. Blanchard D., Diebold B., Peronneau P., Foult J.M., Nee M., Guermonprez J.L., Maurice P.: Non-invasive diagnosis of mitral regurgitation by Doppler echocardiography. Br. Heart J. 1981; 45: 589-593.

33b. Areias J.C., Goldberg S.J., de Villeneuve V.H.: Use and limitations of time interval histogram output from echo Doppler to detect mitral regurgitation. Am. Heart J. 1981; 101: 805-809.

34. Matsuo H., Kitabatake A., Hayashi T., Asao M., Terao Y., Senda S., Hamanaka Y., Matsumoto M., Nimura Y., Abe H.: Intracardiac flow dynamics with bi-directional ultrasound pulsed Doppler technique. Jpn. Circ. J. 1977; 41: 515-528.

35. Miyatake K., Kinoshita N., Nagata S., Beppu S., Park Y., Sakakibara H., Nimura Y.: Intracardiac flow pattern in mitral regurgitation studied with combined use of the ultrasonic pulsed Doppler technique and cross-sectional echocardiography. Am. J. Cardiol. 1980; 45: 155-162.

35a. Kalmanson D., Veyrat C., Abitbol G., Farjon M.: Doppler echocardiography and valvular regurgitation with special emphasis on mitral insufficiency. Advantages of two-dimensional echocardiography with real-time spectral analysis. *In:* Echocardiology. Edited by Rijsterborgh H. Hague, Martinus Nijhoff, 1981; 279-290.

36. Nichol P.M., Boughner D.R., Persaūd J.A.: Noninvasive assessment of mitral regurgitation by trans-cutaneous Doppler ultrasound. Circulation 1976; 54: 656-661.

37. Holen J., Simonsen S., Frøysaker T.: An ultrasound Doppler technique for the noninvasive determination of the pressure gradient in the Bjørk-Shiley mitral valve. Circulation 1979; 59: 436-442.

38. Ubago J.L., Figueroa A., Colman T., Ochoteco A., Duran C.: Hemo-dynamic factors that affect calculated orifice areas in the mitral Hancock xenograft valve. Circulation 1980; 61: 388-394.

39. Alam M., Madrazo A.D., Magilligan D.J., Goldstein S.: M-mode and two-dimensional echocardiographic features of porcine valve dysfunction. Am. J. Cardiol. 1979; 43: 502-509.

40. Harrison E.E., Sbar S., Spoto E., Clark P.: Echocardiogram in porcine mitral valve dysfunction. Am. J. Cardiol. 1980; 45: 908.

41. Levang O.W., Nitter-Hauge S., Levorstad K., Frøysaker T.: Aortic valve replacement. A randomized study comparing the Bjørk-Shiley and Lillehei-Kaster disc valves. Scand. J. Thorac. Cardiovasc. Surg. 1979; 13: 199-213.

42. Hernandez R.R., Greenfield J.C., Mc Call B. W.: Pressure-flow studies in hypertrophic subaortic stenosis. J. Clin. Invest. 1964; 43: 401-407.

43. Pierce G.E., Morrow A.G., Braunwald E.: Idiopathic hypertrophic subaortic stenosis. III. Intraoperative studies of the mechanism of obstruction and its haemodynamic consequences. Circulation 1964; 30 (Suppl. 4): 152-174.
44. Joyner C.R., Harrison F.S., Gruber J.W.: Diagnosis of hypertrophic subaortic stenosis with a Doppler velocity flow detector. Ann. Intern. Med., 1971; 74: 692-696.
45. Boughner D.R., Shield R.L., Persaud J.A.: Hypertrophic obstructive cardiomyopathy. Assessment by echo-cardiographic and Doppler ultrasound techniques. Br. Heart J. 1975; 37: 917-923.
46. Johnson S.L., Baker D.W., Lute R.A., Dodge H.T.: Doppler echo-cardiography. The localization of cardiac murmurs. Circulation 1973; 48: 810-822.
47. Murgo J.P., Alter B.R., Dorethy J.F., Altobelli S.A., Mc Granahan G.M., Dunne T.E.: Dynamics of left ventricular ejection in obstructive and nonobstructive hypertrophic cardiomyopathy. J. Clin. Invest. 1980; 66: 1369-1382.
48. Ambrose J.A., Teichholz L.E., Meller J., Weintraub W., Pichard A.D., Smith H., Martinez E.E., Herman M.V.: The influence of left ventricular late diastolic filling on the A wave of the left ventricular pressure trace. Circulation 1979; 60: 510-519.
48a. Tanouchi J., Inoue M., Kitabatake A., Hori M., Asao M., Mishima M., Shimazu T., Morita H., Masuyama T., Abe H., Matsuo H.: Impaired early diastolic filling of left ventricle in hypertensive patients assessed by intracardiac pulsed Doppler flowmetry. Circulation 1981; 64 (Suppl. IV): 255 (Abstract).
49. Weisfeldt M.L., Fredriksen J.W., Yin F.C., Weiss J.L.: Evidence of incomplete left ventricular relaxation in the dog. Prediction from the time constant for isovolumic pressure fall. J. Clin. Invest. 1978; 62: 1296-1302.
50. Fioretti P., Brower R.W., Maester G.T., Serruys P.W.: Interaction of left ventricular relaxation and filling during early diastole in human subjects. Am. J. Cardiol. 1980; 46: 197-203.
51. Venco A., Recusani F., Sgalambro A.: Diastolic movement of mitral valve in hypertrophic cardiomyopathy. An echocardiographic study. Br. Heart J. 1980; 43: 159-163.
52. Hanrath P., Mathey D.G., Siegert R., Bleifeld W.: Left ventricular relaxation and filling pattern in different forms of left ventricular hypertrophy: An echocardiographic study. Am. J. Cardiol. 1980; 45: 15-23.
53. Sanderson J.E., Traill T.A., Sutton M.G.St J., Brown D.J., Gibson D.G., Goodwin J.F.: Left ventricular relaxation and filling in hypertrophic cardiomyopathy. An echocardiographic study. Br. Heart J. 1978; 40: 596-601.
54. Moreya E., Klein J.J., Shimada H., Segal B.L.: Idiopathic hypertrophic subaortic stenosis diagnosed by reflected ultrasound. Am. J. Cardiol. 1969; 23: 32-37.
55. Stevenson J.G., Kawabori I., Dooley T., Guntheroth W.G.: Diagnosis of ventricular septal defect by pulsed Doppler echocardiography—sensitivity, specificity and limitations. Circulation 1978; 58: 322-326.
56. Magherini A., Azzolina G., Wiechmann V., Fantini F.: Pulsed Doppler echocardiography for diagnosis of ventricular septal defects. Br. Heart J. 1980; 43: 143-147.
57. Hatle L., Rokseth R.: Noninvasive diagnosis and assessment of ventricular septal defect by Doppler ultrasound. Acta Med. Scand. 1981; Suppl. 645: 47-56.
58. Richards K.L., Hockenga D.E., Leach J.K., Blaustein J.C.: Doppler cardiographic diagnosis of interventricular septal rupture. Chest 1979; 76: 101-103.
59. Stevenson J.G., Kawabori I., Guntheroth W.G.: Noninvasive detection of pulmonary hypertension in patent ductus arteriosus by pulsed Doppler echocardiography. Circulation 1979; 60: 355-359.
60. Feldtman R.W., Andrassy R.J., Alexander J.A., Stanford W.: Doppler ultrasonic flow detection as an adjunct in the diagnosis of patent ductus arteriosus in premature infants. J. Thorac. Cardiovasc. Surg. 1976; 72: 288-290.
60a. Stevenson J.G., Kawabori I., Guntheroth W.G.: Pulsed Doppler echocardiographic diagnosis of patent ductus arteriosus: sensitivity, specificity, limitations and technical features. Cathet. Cardiovasc. Diagn. 1980; 6: 255-263.
60b. Allen H.D., Sahn D.J., Lange L., Goldberg S.J.: Noninvasive assessment of surgical systemic to pulmonary artery shunts by range-gated pulsed Doppler echocardiography. J. Pediatr. 1979; 94: 395-402.
60c. Stevenson J.G., Dooley T.K., Kawabori I.: Patent ductus arteriosus in a neonatal intensive care unit: The utility of pulsed Doppler echocardiography. Circulation 1978; 58 (Suppl. III): 110 (Abstract).

60d. Daniels O., Hopman J.C.W., Stoelinga G.B.A., Busch H.J., Peer P.G.M.: A combined Doppler echocardiographic investigation in premature infants with and without respiratory distress syndrome. *In:* Echocardiology. Edited by Rijsterborgh H. Hague, Martinus Nijhoff, 1981; 409-415.

61. Johnson S.L., Rubenstein S., Kawabori I., Dooley D.K., Baker D.W.: The detection of atrial septal defect by pulsed Doppler flowmeter. Circulation 1976; 53-54 (Suppl. II): 168 (Abstract).

62. Goldberg S.J., Areias J.C., Spitaels S.E.C., de Villeneuve V.H.: Use of time interval histographic output from echo-Doppler to detect left-to-right atrial shunts. Circulation 1978; 58: 147-152.

63. Colocousis J.C., Huntsman L.L., Curreri P.W.: Estimation of stroke volume changes by ultrasonic Doppler. Circulation 1977; 56: 914-917.

64. Greenfield J.C., Patel D.J.: Relation between pressure and diameter in the ascending aorta of man. Circ. Res. 1962; 10: 778-781.

65. Hoenecke H.R., Goldberg S.J., Carnahan Y., Sahn D.J., Allen H.D., Valdes-Cruz L.M.: Controlled quantitative assessment of pulmonary and aortic flow by range-gated pulsed Doppler in children with cardiac disease. Circulation 1981; 64 (Suppl. IV): 167 (Abstract).

65a. Berman W., Eldridge M., Yabek S., Dillon T., Alverson D., Rupas D., Bouma K., Hendon L.: Pulsed Doppler determination of cardiac output in neonates and children. Circulation 1981; 64 (Suppl. IV): 167 (Abstract).

65b. Elkayam U., Gardin J., Berkley R., Hughes C., Henry W.L.: The value of aortic blood flow measurements using Doppler technique for the quantitative assessment of changes in stroke volume. Circulation 1981; 64 (Suppl. IV): 256 (Abstract).

66. Magnin P.A., Stewart J.A., Myers S., von Ramm O., Kisslo J.A.: Combined Doppler and phased-array echocardiographic estimation of cardiac output. Circulation 1981; 63: 388-392.

67. Buchtal A., Hanson C., Peisach A.R.: Transcutaneous aortovelography. Potentially useful technique in management of critically ill patients. Br. Heart J. 1976; 38: 451-456.

68. Benchimol A., Barreto E.C., Teng Wei Tio S.: Phasic aortic flow velocity in patients with pulsus alternans. Br. Heart J. 1970; 32: 696-700.

69. Elzinga G., Westerhof N.: Pressure and flow generated by the left ventricle against different impedances. Circ. Res. 1973; 32: 178-186.

69a. Gullace G., Savoia M.T., Ravizza P., Locatelli V., Addamiano P., Ranzi C.: Contrast echocardiographic feature of pulmonary hypertension and regurgitation. Br. Heart J. 1981; 46: 369-373.

69b. Lucas C., Wilcox B., Shallal J., Malouf N.: Pulmonary blood flow wave form in children with ventricular septal defect. World Congress of Pediatric Cardiology, 1980; 290 (Abstract).

69c. Redel D., Victor S.: Pulsed Doppler echocardiography—a noninvasive method for assessment of pulmonary hypertension. World Congress of Pediatric Cardiology, 1980; 323 (Abstract).

70. Murgo J.P., Westerhof N., Giolma J.P., Altobelli S.A.: Manipulation of ascending aortic pressure and flow wave reflections with the Valsalva maneuver: Relationships to input impedance. Circulation 1981; 63: 122-132.

71. Kolettis M., Jenkins B.S., Webb-Pebloe M.M.: Assessment of left ventricular function by indices derived from aortic flow velocity. Br. Heart J. 1976; 38: 18-31.

72. Klinke W.P., Christie L.G., Nichols W.W., Ray M.E., Curry C., Pepine C.J., Conti C.R.: Use of catheter-tip velocity-pressure transducer to evaluate left ventricular function in man: Effects of intravenous propranolol. Circulation 1980; 61: 946-954.

73. Hegrenes L.: Systolic time intervals with Doppler. To be published.

6

*Measurements of High Velocities With Pulsed Doppler**

6.1   INTRODUCTION

The previous chapter discusses how important information can be obtained from measuring maximal blood flow velocities. To be able to measure higher velocities with pulsed Doppler would, therefore, be useful. This would give a better localization of high-velocity jets and make separation of two different high-velocity jets possible or easier. The better signal-to-noise ratio in the pulsed mode could also make recording of weak signals easier.

As described in Section 3.3, higher limits for the velocities that can be recorded in the pulsed mode can be obtained by increasing the pulse repetition rate and/or by using a lower emitted frequency. In addition, the range ambiguity (see Section 3.3) can increase this limit when a pulsed Doppler with changing repetition rates is used. By using a complex spectral analysis of the Doppler signal, one can achieve a doubling of the velocities that can be measured in the pulsed mode (see Sections 3.6 and 8.4C).

The best documentation of a Doppler signal is a recording of the audio signal which contains all the available information. For visual documentation, the spectral analysis shows the distribution of frequencies in the Doppler signal better than the mean and the maximal estimators. This may help later, especially for assessing the quality of a Doppler signal and determining whether velocities may have been underestimated. Spectral analysis might also help when noise may lead to overestimation of velocities (see Figures 5.81 and 5.82). In such cases, a clear border between the noise and the Doppler frequencies may not be possible to obtain even with spectral analysis. The maximal velocity may, therefore, remain uncertain, but a false line would not be recorded as with the estimator.

This chapter describes the recording of high velocities in the pulsed mode using either the mean and maximal estimators or a complex spectral analysis.

*Editors' Note: Kjell Kristoffersen contributed to the writing of this chapter.

6.2   METHODS

The instruments used for the measurements described in this chapter are a combined pulsed and continuous Doppler with frequencies of 1, 2, 5, and 10 MHz* and a complex spectral analyzer as shown in Figure 1.3.† The Doppler has a high maximal pulse repetition rate for use in the near field and a lower one for measurements further from the transducer. They are both continuously variable giving an optimal pulse repetition rate for each depth. The instrument changes frequency automatically when changing transducers. The sample volume for 1 and 2 MHz has a length of approximately 5 mm with the high pulse repetition rate and 10 mm with the low one. The diameter is approximately 5 mm. With 5 MHz, the length is about 2 mm with the high and 4 mm with the low pulse repetition rate. The instrument has a high-pass filter with a continuously variable cut-off frequency of 100 to 1400 Hz.

Figure 6.1A shows the limits for the maximal velocities that can be recorded in the pulsed mode depending on frequency, depth, and a high or low pulse repetition rate. As described in Section 3.3, ambiguity in depth may occur when the pulse repetition rate is so high that the signal from one pulse is not back to the transducer before the next pulse is transmitted. Therefore, the Doppler signal from a certain depth can be recorded both at the correct depth setting and at a lesser depth setting where the signal from the previous pulse is found. The difference in distance between the "real"

*Alfred, Vingmed a/s, Norway.

†Daisy, Vingmed a/s, Norway

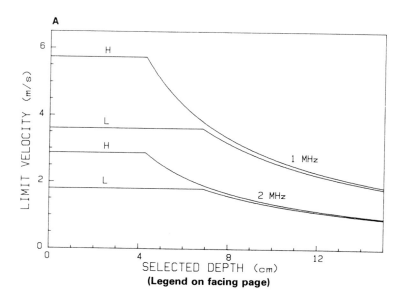

(Legend on facing page)

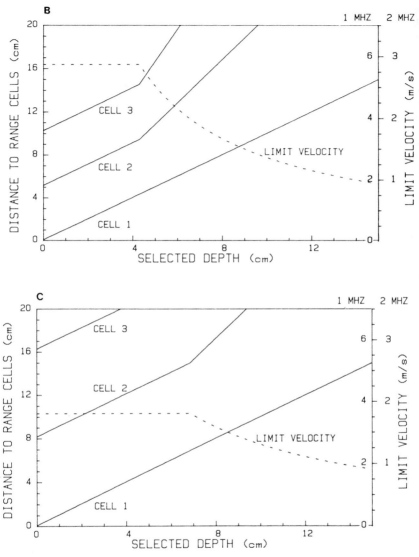

Fig. 6–1. A, The limit velocity of the Alfred instrument in PW mode plotted against the depth settings for the ultrasound carrier frequencies 1 and 2 MHz. For small depth settings, the pulse repetition frequency (PRF) and, thus, the limit velocity are fixed at a maximum value. At larger depth settings the PRF varies continuously with the depth. H—High maximum PRF (14.7 kHz) and high resolution mode. L—Low maximum PRF (9.3 kHz) and low resolution mode. B, Depth ambiguity diagram for Alfred valid in H mode for 1 and 2 MHz. When the selected depth is smaller than 4.5 cm, the distance between the ambiguous range cells is 5.2 cm. The maximum limit velocity is 2.9 m/s for 2 MHz. C, The same diagram as in B valid in the L mode. Here the distance between the range cells is 8.2 cm for small depth settings. The maximum limit velocity is 1.8 m/s with 2 MHz.

and the ambiguous signal depends on the depth and the pulse repetition rate. It is depicted in Figure 6.1B. Since the pulse repetition rate with this Doppler is higher at lesser depth settings, higher velocities can be recorded at a lesser depth setting. By recording the ambiguous signal instead of the real signal, one can obtain a higher velocity in the pulsed mode.

The spectrum analyzer can be set in a mode in which its analyzing range is automatically adjusted to twice the pulse repetition rate of the Doppler instrument. This range can be divided arbitrarily between positive and negative Doppler shifts. Thus, it is possible to use the whole range for velocities in one direction at a time. This enables one to measure velocities twice as high as usual in the pulsed mode, as shown in Figure 6.1. Higher velocities in both directions can be recorded as long as they occur at different times, such as in systole and diastole. Velocities in both directions at the same time cannot be assessed if they are so high that the signals from the two sides of the range mix.

The clinical examination is performed as described in Chapters 4 and 5. The CW mode is used initially to find characteristic or abnormal flow signals or high-velocity jets, then the pulsed mode is used to locate these in depth and in relation to the various valves. For velocities exceeding the limit for the pulsed mode at depths > 6 to 7 cm, the range ambiguity is regularly applied in order to obtain the highest velocity possible in the pulsed mode. By this method, velocities at the mitral and aortic valve areas can often be better recorded at a depth setting of 4 to 5 cm instead of at the real depth of 9 to 12 cm. In most patients, this is easily accomplished since few or no other Doppler signals usually occur at the lesser depth. In patients with very large hearts, however, problems with mixed signals may occur even if the highest velocities are still recorded. A much lower pulse repetition rate can then be used to obtain unambiguous recordings.

For recording velocities in infants or close to the transducer, a frequency of 5 MHz is used. Otherwise, the 2 MHz is most frequently used, except for high velocities at larger depths where 1 MHz must be applied to record these in the pulsed mode.

Mean and maximal velocities are recorded together with the amplitude of the Doppler signal, the ECG and the phonocardiogram, and an ordinary paper recorder (Elema Mingograph). The spectral curve is recorded together with the amplitude, ECG, and phonocardiogram on a grey-scale line-scan recorder (Tektronix).

6.3   CLINICAL APPLICATIONS

Use of the range ambiguity to obtain a higher velocity in the pulsed mode is shown in Figure 6.2. The patient was a three-year-old child seen following operation for Fallot's tetralogy. Both infundibular and valvular obstruction had been present before operation. A maximal velocity of 4.6 m/s and an

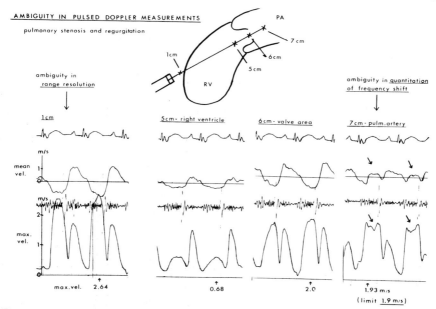

Fig. 6–2. Pulmonary stenosis and regurgitation recorded with 2 MHz pulsed Doppler. In the right ventricle velocity is normal in systole and pulmonary regurgitation is seen toward the transducer in diastole. At the valve area velocity in systole is increased and just above the valve it is seen to exceed the limit for the pulsed mode at this depth. At 1 cm depth the higher velocity above the valve could be recorded.

increased velocity at infundibular level had been recorded with CW Doppler. Postoperatively, an increased velocity which exceeded the limit for the pulsed mode was found at the orifice and just above the valve (Figure 6.2, 7 cm). The valve area was just far enough away from the transducer to make it possible to record the previous pulse from this area closer to the transducer (1 cm). The velocity of 2.6 m/s was within the limit for the 2 MHz frequency of this depth, and the distortions of the mean velocity curve at 7 cm were no longer present. Thus, the range ambiguity could be used to avoid ambiguity in quantitation of the frequency shift.

The use of a lower frequency to record higher velocities in the pulsed mode is shown in Figure 6.3. In a patient with VSD, a high-velocity jet toward the transducer in the third left intercostal space was recorded from 2 to 4 cm depth. Velocity at 4 cm depth was above the limit for the pulsed mode with 2 MHz and too close to the transducer to make use of the range ambiguity. With 1 MHz, a velocity of 4.35 m/s was recorded and a pressure drop of 75 mm Hg from the left to the right ventricle was calculated. The systolic blood pressure was 100 mm Hg, and right ventricular systolic pressure was, therefore, within normal range. That this high velocity was within

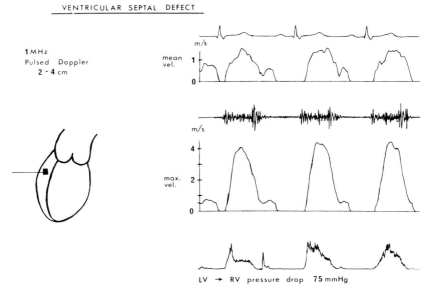

Fig. 6–3. **A high-velocity jet toward the transducer between 2 and 4 cm depth was recorded from the third left intercostal space in a child with VSD. The velocity at 4 cm depth exceeded the limit for 2 MHz so a frequency of 1 MHz had to be used. A pressure drop of 75 mm Hg between the two ventricles was calculated. Tricuspid flow velocity toward the transducer in diastole with tricuspid valve opening in the first beat shows the sample volume to be in the right ventricle. The low velocity of tricuspid flow following atrial contraction is not shown because a high filter setting is used to improve the recording of the high velocity.**

the right ventricle was shown by the simultaneous recording of tricuspid flow velocities in diastole. The ability to record the high-velocity jets in VSD with pulsed Doppler could make it easier to detect the presence of more than one defect in the ventricular septum. This is often impossible using the CW mode, at least in the smaller children and infants. With the larger depth of the mitral orifice in an adult, both the 1 MHz frequency and the range ambiguity had to be used to obtain the increased forward flow velocity and the high velocity in the regurgitant jet in a patient with combined mitral stenosis and regurgitation (Figure 6.4). Whereas the use of the 1 MHz frequency may give inferior Doppler signals when blood flow is normal or when only low velocities are present, the signals obtained from higher velocities are as good or better than those obtained with a higher frequency. The ability to record both forward and regurgitant flow velocities at the valve area with the pulsed mode and without frequency aliasing (see Section 3.6) might increase the possibilities of quantitating the regurgitant flow.

Figure 6.5 illustrates how the spectral analyzer is used to increase the velocities that can be recorded in the pulsed mode. In this patient with mitral stenosis and regurgitation, CW Doppler gave a maximal velocity of 2 m/s in

MITRAL STENOSIS AND REGURGITATION

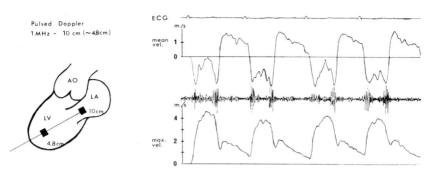

Fig. 6–4. In a patient with mitral stenosis and regurgitation both a frequency of 1 MHz and the range ambiguity were necessary to record the high velocities at the mitral orifice in the pulsed mode.

the forward flow and 5.5 m/s in the regurgitation. The zero line can be moved as shown in the figure to obtain higher velocities in one direction. High velocities in the opposite direction can also be recorded as long as they occur at a different time, as depicted in Figure 6.5. The lower velocity of the mitral regurgitation following a short R-R interval reflects the lower systolic

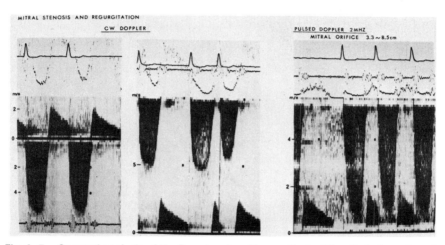

Fig. 6–5. Spectral analysis of the Doppler signal in a patient with mitral stenosis and regurgitation. The increased velocity of forward mitral flow is seen above the zero line and the regurgitation below. If the zero line is moved to one side of the possible range, higher velocities in both directions can be recorded as long as they occur at different times. Flow away from the transducer is now seen from the upper limit of the range. To the right a recording with the pulsed mode from the mitral orifice is shown. When both the range ambiguity and the doubling of the velocity limit with the spectral analyzer are used, a velocity of 5.3 m/s is obtained with pulsed Doppler and a 2 MHz frequency. ECG, phonocardiogram, and the amplitude of the Doppler signal are also shown.

pressure in the left ventricle during this beat. Changing to the pulsed mode, locating the mitral orifice, and using the range ambiguity allowed a velocity of 5.3 m/s to be recorded with a frequency of 2 MHz in the pulsed mode from the mitral regurgitation, as well as a maximal velocity of 2 m/s from the forward mitral flow.

Figure 6.6, which is from the same patient, shows how the regurgitant mitral jet can be followed backward in the left atrium from the mitral orifice at 8 cm to a depth of 15.5 cm indicating a large left atrium. With 2 MHz and without the use of the range ambiguity, the maximal velocity in the regurgitant jet exceeds the limit for the pulsed mode. The Doppler signal from the regurgitation is strongest at the mitral valve area and just behind, and it gradually weakens from 3 cm behind the valve and further back in the left atrium. This can be seen from both the spectrum and the amplitude curve. To be able to record the regurgitant flow as far back as it extends, one must first find the best direction to the regurgitation with CW Doppler.

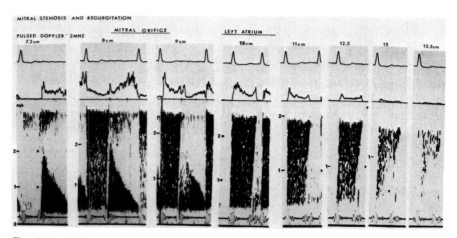

Fig. 6–6. ECG, amplitude and spectrum of Doppler signal, and phonocardiogram in a patient with mitral stenosis and regurgitation. The forward mitral flow (toward the transducer) is seen above the zero line, the regurgitation extending downward from the upper end of the range. When the mitral regurgitation is followed backward in the left atrium, a strong Doppler signal is found at the mitral valve area and for 2 to 3 cm behind the valve. Further back the signal becomes gradually weaker, shown by both the spectral curve and the amplitude.

In hypertrophic obstructive cardiomyopathy, the ability to record higher velocities in the pulsed mode has made it possible to distinguish between the high-velocity jet from an intraventricular obstruction and that of the associated mitral regurgitation. This allows one to record the maximal velocity within the left ventricle and to assess the degree of intraventricular obstruction. In the patient shown in Figure 6.7, velocity in the left ventricle in systole

HYPERTROPHIC OBSTRUCTIVE CARDIOMYOPATHY

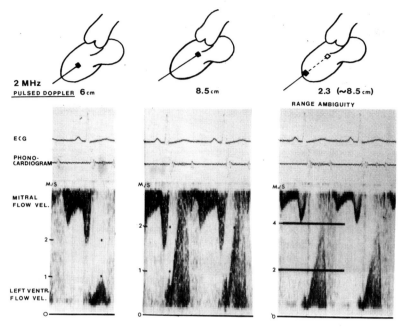

Fig. 6–7. The polarity of the Doppler signal was changed in this patient showing the velocity in the left ventricle in systole from the zero line and the mitral flow velocity from the upper end of the range. Increase in velocity in systole from 6 to 8.5 cm depth is seen, and use of the range ambiguity shows a maximal velocity of 4 m/s. The increase in mitral flow velocity following atrial contraction is pronounced.

was normal at 6 cm depth. At 8.5 cm, a marked increase exceeding the limit for the pulsed mode was found. When the range ambiguity was used, a maximal velocity of 4 m/s was recorded, indicating a pressure drop of 64 mm Hg within the left ventricle. The late systolic maximum of the flow velocity is characteristic of a dynamic obstruction. Forward mitral flow velocity with a marked increase following atrial contraction is seen from the upper end of the range in this patient, as polarity can be changed for easier measurement of the velocity of main interest.

The distance between the mitral regurgitation at the mitral valve area and the intraventricular obstruction is very small due to small left ventricular cavities in these patients. Therefore, even when recording in the pulsed mode, one has to be careful to separate these lesions. The velocity patterns, however, differ clearly. Rise of velocity in the left ventricle is later and slower, while the velocity of the mitral regurgitation is high from the beginning due to the large left ventricular-left atrial pressure difference. This difference can be seen when comparing Figures 6.6, 6.7, and 6.9.

Figure 6.8, which is from another patient with hypertrophic obstructive cardiomyopathy, shows increase in velocity in the left ventricle between 6 and 7 cm depth. A premature beat with increase in velocity is presumably due to decreased ventricular filling and increased obstruction.

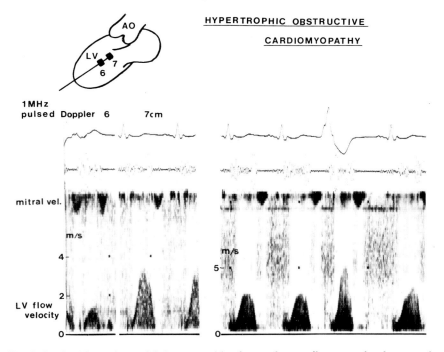

Fig. 6–8.   In this patient with hypertrophic obstructive cardiomyopathy, increase in velocity was found between 6 and 7 cm depth, and a clear increase in velocity in premature beats was consistently found. With the 1 MHz frequency, the high velocity at this depth could be recorded without use of the range ambiguity.

Figures 6.9 and 6.10 are from the same patient. Despite the presence here of several lesions in one patient, the lesions can be separated and assessed with the present technique. Figure 6.9 depicts how the Doppler signal may improve with slight changes in direction and how well this is seen in the spectral curve, as shown for mitral flow velocity from A and B to C. Because the mitral regurgitation was very mild in this patient, a better recording of the regurgitation was not obtained, but the difference between the regurgitation and left ventricular systolic flow velocity is still clear. The late systolic increase in velocity seen at 8 cm depth in Figure 6.10 is the characteristic pattern observed with cavity obliteration, and an obstruction above this level may or may not be present. This patient had a significant subvalvular obstruction due to pronounced left ventricular hypertrophy that had produced

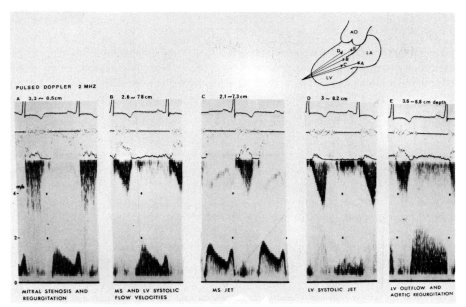

Fig. 6-9. The velocity curves are from different positions in the left ventricle and the mitral valve area in a patient with mitral stenosis and regurgitation, and subvalvular and aortic valve stenosis and regurgitation. Velocities toward the transducer are seen above the zero line, whereas velocities away are seen from the top of the spectral display extending downward. A is from the mitral orifice and shows the mitral stenosis and regurgitation. B shows flow velocity in the left ventricle in systole. Note the difference between the two systolic flow patterns. C and D show that when the transducer is directed more toward the mitral orifice (C) or the left ventricular outflow tract (D), better Doppler signals with fewer low frequencies are obtained from the diastolic (C) and systolic (D) flow. In E aortic regurgitation is shown, but the spectral curve with mostly low frequencies indicates a substantial angle to both systolic and regurgitant flow.

a narrow subaortic tunnel. The calculated subvalvular pressure drop was 67 mm Hg. The higher maximal velocity recorded from above (first right intercostal space) might be due to a better angle to this velocity or to an additional pressure drop across the aortic valve. At catheterization, a peak pressure drop of 78 mm Hg was recorded below the aortic valve. Moderate aortic regurgitation and mitral stenosis as well as a very mild mitral regurgitation were also present.

The ability to record high velocities with pulsed Doppler has also made it possible to estimate the length of poststenotic jets. In an experimental study using carbon particles to visualize the flow through and past obstructions, a jet length of 12 to 15 mm was found with a post-jet flow disturbance of 40 to 46 mm.[1] When jet velocities in aortic and mitral stenosis were recorded with the pulsed Doppler described in this chapter, the maximal velocities

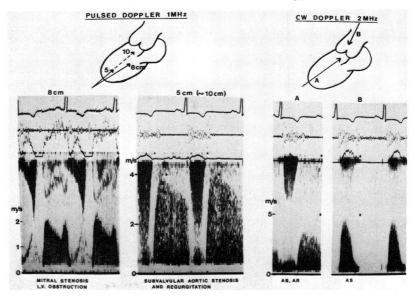

Fig. 6–10. A recording from the same patient as in Figure 6.9 shows at 8 cm a mainly late systolic increase in velocity, whereas 2 cm higher up in the outflow tract increase in velocity is larger and is also found earlier in systole. Maximal velocity recorded below the aortic valve was 4.1 m/s indicating a subvalvular pressure drop of 67 mm Hg. With CW Doppler from above, a maximal velocity of 4.7 m/s was recorded with a calculated pressure drop of 88 mm Hg, while from below, velocity was comparable to that obtained with the pulsed mode.

recorded at the orifice could be found up to 4 cm from the orifice. Thereafter, a gradual decrease in velocity occurred. The Doppler signal at the orifice contains mostly high frequencies, but from 1 to 2 cm a gradual increase of lower frequencies in the signal occurs illustrating the gradual dispersion of the jet.

In Figure 6.11 a pulsed Doppler recording from the mitral jet shows that the increase of lower frequencies/velocities in the sample volume occurs close to the orifice, while even 4 cm from the orifice the decrease in maximal velocity is only moderate. The presence of high velocities for a considerable distance from the orifice explains why it is often easier to record a jet with Doppler than to obtain a cross-sectional valve area with 2-D echocardiography.

In ventricular septal defects, especially in small children, a high-velocity jet may have a shorter distance to disperse, which may explain the pronounced flow disturbance usually found in VSD when there is a significant pressure drop across the septum. By using spectral analysis as well as pulsed Doppler and a filter with a higher cut-off frequency, one can record higher velocities in a larger number of patients with VSD than reported earlier.[2]

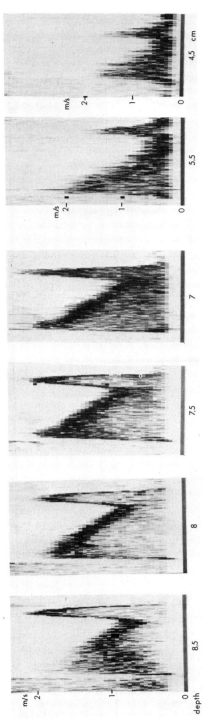

Fig. 6–11. Pulsed Doppler recording from the apex of the mitral jet in a patient with mitral stenosis in sinus rhythm. At the orifice (8 cm) the pure high frequency signal shows as a narrow band of high frequencies throughout diastole. At 8.5 cm the increased velocity is best recorded during atrial contraction while the highest velocities are not yet present in the first part of diastole. This is a usual finding and may be caused by the movement of the heart during diastole so the sample volume is more on the atrial side of the orifice early in diastole than later. When one records closer to the transducer (7.5 to 4.5 cm), an increasing amount of lower frequencies are present in the signal, but high frequencies are still present (note the difference in scale at 5.5 and 4.5 cm).

183

Therefore, failure to record a high velocity present in VSD is probably more often due to the pronounced flow disturbance than to lack of a small enough angle.

6.4 CONCLUSION

As described in Chapter 5 and in this chapter, much hemodynamic information can be obtained from measurements of blood flow velocities in the heart with Doppler ultrasound. With the ability to record higher velocities in the pulsed mode, more information can be obtained.

The main advantage has been a better localization of high-velocity jets and better separation of flow signals when more than one obstruction or high velocity jet have been present. Another advantage is that weak high-frequency signals sometimes are easier to record in the pulsed mode, most likely owing to a better signal-to-noise ratio. In addition, whether the pulsed or the CW mode has to be used, having a filter with a higher cut-off frequency (1400 vs. 900 Hz) in some cases helps one to record a weak signal with high frequencies.

Another possible advantage of recording high velocities in the pulsed mode is that it may improve assessments of valvular regurgitation and make quantitation possible.

One advantage of adding spectral analysis is that a doubling of the limits of the maximal velocity can be obtained. It may also help in assessing the quality of a Doppler signal, and it gives a better visual documentation. In addition, one avoids estimator artifacts due to noise. In most heart lesions, however, the results obtained with the techniques as described in Chapter 5 and in this chapter are similar.

REFERENCES

1. Kececioglu-Draelos Z., Goldberg S.J., Areias J., Sahn D.J.: Verification and clinical demonstration of the echo Doppler series effect and vortex shed distance. Circulation 1981; 63: 1422-1428.
2. Hatle L., Rokseth R.: Noninvasive diagnosis and assessment of ventricular septal defect by Doppler ultrasound. Acta Med. Scand. 1981; Suppl. 645: 47-56.

7

Pulsed Doppler Ultrasound for Measuring Blood Flow in the Human Aorta

Alf O. Brubakk and Svein E. Gisvold

7.1 INTRODUCTION

An easy-to-use, noninvasive, and reliable method for measuring heart function would be of considerable value in many clinical situations. The main criterion for the overall function of the heart is its ability to deliver sufficient blood flow to meet the demands of the peripheral circulation.

By means of echocardiographic methods, aortic blood flow can be calculated indirectly.[1] Because these calculations are based on certain assumptions about left ventricular geometry, however, errors can be introduced if the ventricle is not contracting uniformly, as is often the case in coronary heart disease.[2]

Ultrasound and the Doppler principle show promise of being a technique that offers the possibility of measuring both instantaneous and mean flow in the aorta noninvasively. Both continuous and pulsed ultrasonic Doppler systems can be used. Continuous wave ultrasound, as used by several authors,[3-5] is a simple technique; however, since no range resolution is possible, all velocity signals in the beam are recorded. We have used a pulsed Doppler system with a narrow beam, described in Section 3.3, thus permitting measurement at selected points and avoiding contamination from neighboring arteries and veins. Furthermore, using mean- and maximum-frequency estimators instead of displaying the whole frequency spectrum simplifies the measurement procedure. This is described in more detail in Sections 3.3 and 3.4.

7.2 MEASUREMENT TECHNIQUE

Flow velocity in the aorta can be measured most conveniently from the suprasternal notch, as demonstrated in Figure 7.1. By moving the transducer, one can record the velocities in the ascending aorta and in the aortic arch.

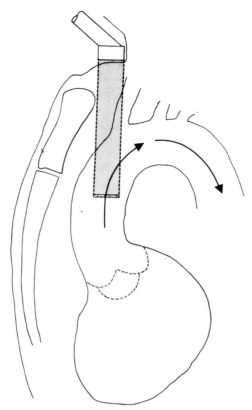

Fig. 7–1. Transducer position in the suprasternal notch for measuring blood flow velocity in the ascending aorta.

We prefer measuring in the ascending aorta, although adequate signals can be obtained from the aortic arch in many subjects. In a normal adult, adequate signals are usually found at distances 5 to 7 cm below the skin surface. In some subjects it can be extremely difficult to obtain adequate signals. This is usually the case in elderly somewhat obese subjects, when the neck is short and the sternum thick. In our experience it is usually easier to obtain adequate signals with the subject supine, although measurements can also be performed with the patient sitting or standing. If the subject is sitting, better signals can usually be obtained by letting him lean slightly forward.

It is important to exert enough pressure on the probe in the dorsal direction. Transducers that are too large do not permit proper measurement in the ascending aorta. A specially designed suprasternal notch transducer with a diameter of 12 mm* was used in Figure 7.1.

*Vingmed a/s, Oslo, Norway

On most occasions, the mean- and maximum-frequency estimators are used and the curves are recorded on an ink-jet recorder. Proper setting of the gain-control is necessary in order to ensure adequate signals.

Adequate Doppler signals can only be obtained if the ultrasonic beam is properly aimed and the sample volume is wholly placed inside the aorta. Figure 7.2 illustrates an example of good-quality signals from the ascending aorta and the aortic arch. The mean and maximum velocities are very close together, indicating a flat cross section of the velocity profile. The presence of a narrow frequency band can also be ascertained by listening to the Doppler shift. Adequate signals have a high frequency whistling sound and, thus, a whistling sound signifies that the sample volume is placed wholly inside the aorta.

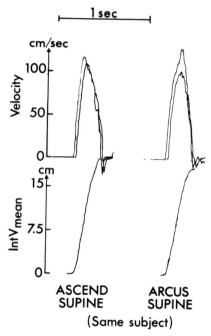

Fig. 7–2. Normal blood flow velocity in signals from the ascending aorta and the aortic arch. Upper panel shows maximal and mean velocities; lower panel shows integral of mean velocity.

If the sample volume is placed partly outside the vessel, the mean velocity will be considerably underestimated as can be seen from Figure 7.3. The difference between mean and maximum velocity can thus be used for judging the quality of the signals. Mean velocity must not be less than 80% of maximum velocity during systole in signals that are to be used for flow calculations.[6]

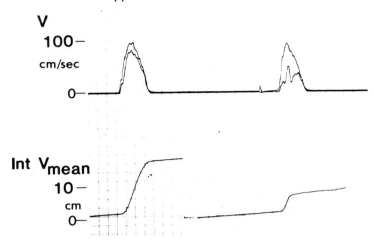

Fig. 7–3.   Reduction in mean flow velocity caused by placing the sample volume partly outside the vessel.

As illustrated in Figure 7.3, maximum velocities are less affected by errors in aiming than mean velocities. However, turbulence and flow disturbances can lead to large local increases in maximum velocities. Values of flow based on maximum velocities are therefore overestimated. Such local velocity disturbances most likely occur close to the aortic valves, but as turbulence can be present in the aorta of man during systole,[7] particularly during the deacceleration phase,[8] local velocity gradients and hence large differences between mean and maximum velocities can sometimes be observed along the whole ascending aorta. In addition, rotating eddies are sometimes found toward end-systole close to the aortic valves.

Proper setting of estimator gain is necessary to obtain adequate signals. Figure 7.4 illustrates the effect of having a too-large gain on the maximum frequency estimator. Maximum velocity will be overestimated (see Section 3.5).

As shown from these examples, both under- and overestimation of mean velocity can occur, and considerable care must be taken when this method is used for calculating velocity and flow.

Two additional points can be made. If changes in blood flow velocities are to be studied, it is important that the measurements are performed at the same depth because changing the sample volume position might change the angle between the ultrasonic beam and the bloodstream. In Figure 7.5, which shows an example of this, the angle at a greater depth is significantly smaller than that found at a shorter distance below the skin. Secondly, each measurement must have sufficient duration in order to eliminate errors due to respiration. During deep respiratory movements, changes in flow up to 30% have been noted.[6]

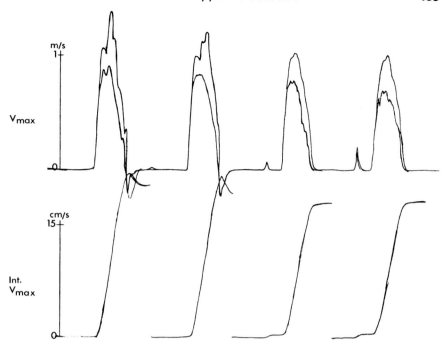

Fig. 7–4. Overestimation of maximal blood flow velocity due to too large gain on maximal velocity estimator.

7.3   CALCULATION OF FLOW AND FLOW VELOCITY

With the instrument used (see Sections 3.3 and 3.4), the following variables can be measured: mean and maximum velocities, integral under the mean- and maximum-velocity curve, acceleration of mean and maximum velocity.

For calculating absolute values of velocity, the angle between the ultrasonic beam and the bloodstream is important. (see Section 3.3). In an earlier study,[9] it was found that the angle between the ultrasonic beam and the bloodstream in the ascending aorta showed considerable variation from person to person (30° to 70°). A later study indicated that a much smaller angle between the beam and velocity direction can be obtained.[6] The reason for this discrepancy is probably that the use of a larger transducer in the first study made access to the ascending aorta at a small angle difficult. Using a special suprasternal notch transducer (diameter approximately 12 mm) and exerting sufficient pressure in the dorsal direction, one can obtain a small angle. When the angle is small, we can approximate it to zero. Figure 7.6 shows the error obtained as a function of the actual angle between the beam

ASCENDING AORTA

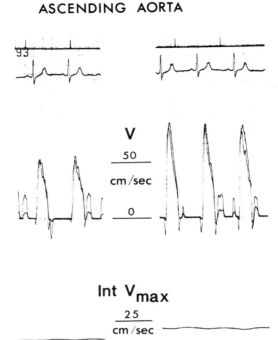

3.5 cm   7.2 cm

Fig. 7–5. Changes in measured blood flow velocity due to difference in sampling depth.

and the velocity direction. Acceleration is a good parameter for judging left ventricular contractile properties.[10] However, in our experience it is often difficult to obtain reproducible and accurate estimates of acceleration from ultrasonic Doppler measurements.

To calculate flow from velocity measurements, the cross-sectional area of the aorta must be known (see Section 2.1). Because this area varies with age and body size, it must be measured if accurate estimates of flow are to be made. This can be done from M-mode measurements of aortic diameter assuming a circular cross section of the aorta is present. The diameter measurement must be accurate since the area is obtained by squaring the diameter. Therefore, the relative inaccuracy in area is twice the relative inaccuracy in diameter. Owing to the elasticity in the aortic wall, the diameter of the aorta varies during systole approximately 15% from the increase in aortic pressure. Therefore, a mean diameter must be used. The diameter

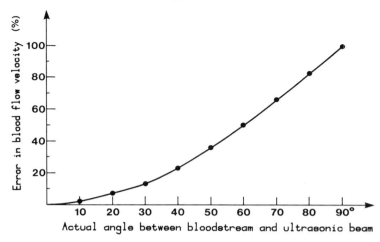

Fig. 7–6. **Error in blood flow velocity estimate (%) plotted against actual angle between bloodstream and ultrasonic beam.**

should also be measured at the location of velocity measurements, which is difficult. The circular shape of aorta is an assumption which may also cause additional error.

Because of the difficulty in obtaining the area and the angle, absolute measurements of volumetric flow rate in the aorta are difficult to obtain with acceptable accuracy. However, for recording relative changes in the flow, we can use the Doppler shift directly without making corrections for angle and area.

The mean velocity over the cross-sectional area is proportional to flow. However, this measure is more sensitive to errors in aiming than maximum velocity. Furthermore, interference from other vessels might reduce the mean velocity. Maximum velocity is less sensitive to aiming because the velocity profile in the aorta is fairly flat (see Section 2.3). It should, therefore, be preferable for calculating changes in flow. However, several theoretical problems exist regarding the maximum velocity estimator, particularly in relation to the definition of the maximum frequencies present (see Section 3.5B). No firm advice can be offered regarding which of the two mentioned variables is better for calculating relative changes in flow, but as long as only signals where mean and maximum velocity are close to each other are used, each of them should be equally helpful.

From Table 7·1 the reproducibility of the method can be judged. The data come from four separate studies performed over shorter or longer periods of time. The operators participating in the two last studies were considerably less skilled than the operators in the first two studies.

Table 7·1   Reproducibility of Doppler Measurements in the Ascending Aorta

	No. of Subjects	No. of Measurements in Each Subject	Time Between Measurements	Mean Variation Coefficient (%)
I.	5	10	days to months	
V_{max}				6.4
Int V_{max}				9.1
Accel				8.6
V mean				9.2
Int V mean				11.7
II.	16	5	minutes	
V_{max}				5.9
Int V_{max}				6.7
Accel				15.1
III.	6	3	minutes	
V_{max}				9.2
Int V_{max}				14.9
IV.	6	3	days	
V_{max}				9.7
Int V_{max}				16.5

Table 7·2   Ascending Aortic Velocities in the Supine Position (Mean Values ± SD)

	Males	Females
No. of Subjects	14	13
I. V_{max} (cm/sec)	119 ± 12.0	108 ± 8.7
Int V_{max} (cm)	20.2 ± 2.1	19.2 ± 2.1
No. of Subjects	15	
II. V_{max} (cm/sec)	106 ± 7.0	
Int V_{max} (cm)	16 ± 3.0	

Table 7·2 shows values of maximum velocity and integral under the velocity curve found in healthy subjects in two separate studies.

From these data it seems reasonable to conclude that changes in flow and flow velocity of 20 to 25% can be detected.

REFERENCES

1. Murray J.A., Johnston W., Reid J.M.: Echocardiographic determination of left ventricular dimensions, volumes and performance. Am. J. Cardiol. 1972; 30: 252-257.

44444444

444444444

4444444444

2. Teichholz L.E., Kreulen T.H., Herman W.V., Gorlin R.: Problems in echocardiographic volume determination. Circulation 1972; 46 Suppl 2: 75 (abstract).
3. Light L.H.: Noninjurious ultrasonic technique for observing flow in the human aorta. Nature 1969; 224: 1119-1121.
4. Mackay R.S.: Non-invasive cardiac output measurement. Microvasc. Res. 1972; 4: 438-452.
5. Huntsman L.L., Gams E., Johnson C.C., Fairbanks E.: Transcutaneous determination of aortic blood flow velocities in man. Am. Heart J. 1975; 89: 605-612.
6. Gisvold S.E., Brubakk A.O.: Measurement of instantaneous blood-flow velocity in the human aorta using pulsed ultrasound. Cardiovasc. Res. In press, 1982.
7. Stein D.D., Sabbak H.N.: Turbulent blood-flow in the ascending aorta of humans with normal and diseased aortic valves. Circ. Res. 1976; 39: 58-65.
8. Schultz D.L., Tunstall-Pedoe D.S., Lee G. de J., Gunning A.J., Bellhouse B.J.: Velocity distribution and transition in the arterial system. In: Ciba Foundation Symposium on Circulatory and Respiratory Mass Transport, London, Churchill, 1969; 172-199.
9. Angelsen B., Brubakk A.O.: Transcutaneous measurement of blood-flow velocity in the human aorta. Cardiovasc. Res. 1976; 10: 368-379.
10. Noble M.I.M., Trenchard D., Guz A.: Left ventricular ejection in conscious dogs. Circ. Res. 1966; 19: 139-152.

8

Spectrum Analysis

8.1 INTRODUCTION

Spectrum analysis is a central topic in ultrasonic Doppler blood velocity measurements. The reason for this is, of course, that the velocity of the scatterer is coded into the scattered wave as a change in frequency, the Doppler shift. This is discussed in Chapter 3.

However, our definition of frequency has been nonspecific. In Section 3.4A, it is indicated that the signal from a single scatterer is not a sharp frequency but a distribution of frequencies. This concept is discussed in depth in this chapter. Different concepts of frequency are presented, and the frequency concept which is adequate for our purpose is discussed.

What we want to measure is velocity. In principle, this can be accomplished without the intermediate step of performing spectrum analysis. However, as is discussed in the following section, all information in the Doppler signal is contained in the power spectrum of the signal. Spectrum analysis is, therefore, a convenient way to extract information.

8.2 WHAT IS FREQUENCY?

In the following two sections, we discuss different frequency concepts and conclude that the frequency obtained from Fourier analysis is the relevant concept for Doppler signal analysis.

A. The Fourier Transform and Other Frequency Concepts

Most people have an *intuitive* concept of the frequency of an event as the number of occurrences in a defined interval of time. For example, the frequency of car accidents in a city can be 43 per day or the frequency of heartbeats can be 66 per minute.

This intuitive concept forms the basis of a more rigorous definition of frequency for signals. A signal is called *periodic* with period, T, if it repeats itself after a time, T. The *fundamental* frequency of a periodic signal we then define as

$$f = \frac{1}{T} \qquad (8.1)$$

Fundamental angular frequency is obtained by multiplying by 2π:

$$\omega = 2\pi f = \frac{2\pi}{T} \qquad (8.2)$$

We note that a strictly periodic signal has an *infinite duration* in time; otherwise, there would exist a time limit, after which the signal would not repeat itself.

The Doppler signal from a single scatterer is a burst of oscillations with a finite duration in time, as already discussed in Section 3.4A. The duration of the burst is the transit time, T_t, of the scatterer

$$T_t = \frac{L}{v} \qquad (8.3)$$

where L is the path length of the scatterer through the range cell, and v is the scatterer velocity. Upon demodulation, which we discuss in Section 8.3, the single scatterer signal is

$$x(t) = u(t)\cos\omega_d t \qquad (8.4)$$

where $\omega_d = 2\pi f_d$ and f_d is the Doppler shift given in Equation 3.5. The amplitude of the oscillation is represented by u(t). This signal is shown in Figure 8.1a where u(t) has a rectangular form. From the zero crossings of the signal we can determine f_d:

$$f_d = \frac{1}{T_d} \qquad (8.5)$$

That is, we can determine the velocity exactly from the zero crossings of the signal. The burst in Figure 8.1a is termed *semiperiodic*. There is a certain repetitiveness within the burst, namely the oscillations with period T_d. Since the signal is of finite duration in time, however, it is not strictly periodic according to the preceding discussion. For such a semiperiodic signal, we define the *zero-crossing frequency* as $f_d = T_d^{-1}$.

When the Doppler signal is composed of the sum of the contributions from a large number of scatterers, as in blood velocity measurements, the situation is more complicated. Such a signal is shown in Figure 8.1b. Neither of the aforementioned frequency definitions applies to this signal. A frequency

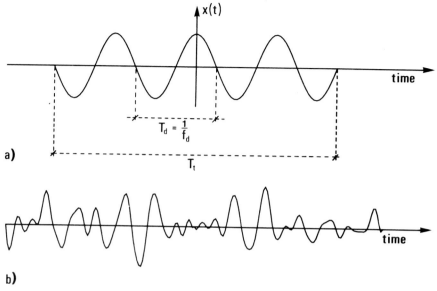

Fig. 8–1. **a) Doppler signal from single scatterer. b) Composite Doppler signal from many scatterers.**

definition that can be used in this situation is obtained from the Fourier transform.[1] Let $x(t)$ denote the signal. Its Fourier transform, $X(\omega)$, is then defined as

$$X(\omega) = \int_{-\infty}^{\infty} dt\ x(t)\ e^{-i\omega t} \tag{8.6}$$

The signal itself can be obtained from its Fourier transform as

$$x(t) = \frac{1}{2\pi} \int_{-\infty}^{\infty} d\omega\ X(\omega)\ e^{i\omega t} \tag{8.7}$$

The variable ω is called the *angular Fourier frequency* for reasons which are discussed subsequently. The *Fourier frequency* is obtained by dividing by 2π: $f = \omega/2\pi$. The Fourier transform, $X(\omega)$, is sometimes called the *Fourier spectrum* or *Fourier frequency distribution*.

   The Fourier transform of the single scatterer Doppler signal in Figure 8.1a is shown in Figure 8.2, where $\omega_d = 2\pi f_d$ is the *Doppler angular frequency*. The Fourier transform presents a *distribution* of Fourier frequencies, both positive and negative. Two main lobes are centered at $\pm\ \omega_d$, and there are several side lobes. The width of the main lobes is

$$\triangle\omega_d = \frac{2\pi}{T_t} \tag{8.8}$$

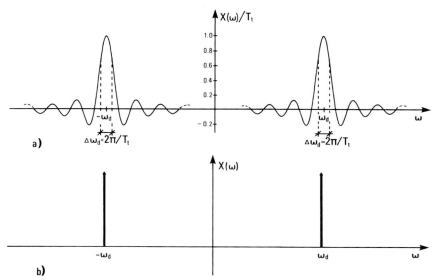

Fig. 8–2. Fourier transform of cosine burst (a) and infinite cosine wave (b).

When the length of the burst increases, the width of the main lobes decreases. As $T_t \to \infty$, the Fourier transform tends toward two spikes at $\pm\, \omega_d$ as illustrated in Figure 8.2b.

Thus, for an infinite cosine train, the Fourier transform gives the same frequency that is obtained from the inverse distance between zero crossings in Figure 8.1a.

There is also both a *positive* and a *negative* component. This is a purely mathematical result from the definition of the complex exponential term

$$e^{i\omega t} = \cos\omega t + i\sin\omega t \qquad\qquad (8.9)$$

which gives

$$\cos\omega t = \frac{1}{2}\{e^{i\omega t} + e^{-i\omega t}\} \qquad (8.10a)$$

$$(8.10)$$

$$\sin\omega t = \frac{1}{2i}\{e^{i\omega t} - e^{-i\omega t}\} \qquad (8.10b)$$

Cos ωt and sin ωt are represented by both $+\omega t$ and $-\omega t$ in the exponential portion of the equation.

For physical waveforms, the positive and negative frequencies combine to produce a real signal. If x (t) is a complex signal, there is no such relationship between positive and negative frequencies, a situation which we shall use in the analysis of Doppler signals in Sections 8.3 and 8.4C.

We now return to the case where T_t is finite in Figure 8.1a. The maximum of the Fourier frequency distribution gives the zero-crossing frequency of the burst, which in turn gives the scatterer velocity. However, if noise is present in the signal, we obtain a corroboration of the Fourier transform in Figure 8.2a. This introduces an uncertainty in the determination of ω_d from the Fourier spectrum. This uncertainty depends on the signal-to-noise power ratio (S/N ratio). In addition, in the general situation when the signal is composed of more than one burst, the zero-crossing frequencies of the bursts must be some distance apart in order to separate the main lobes from the different bursts in the spectrum.

Both these situations introduce an uncertainty in determining the zero-crossing frequency from the Fourier spectrum. The uncertainty in angular zero-crossing frequency is approximately the width of the main lobe

$$\triangle \omega_d = \frac{2\pi}{T_t} \tag{8.11}$$

or in terms of frequency

$$\triangle f_d = \frac{1}{T_t} \tag{8.12}$$

That is, the accuracy by which we can determine the Doppler shift of a scatterer using Fourier methods is inversely proportional to the transit time. Using Equation 8.3 for T_t and Equation 3.5 for the relationship between f_d and v, we find that Equation 8.12 takes the form

$$\frac{\triangle f_d}{f_d} = \frac{\lambda}{2L\cos\theta}$$

which is the same as Equation 3.9.

A signal can in general be written in the form

$$\mathbf{x(t) = a(t) \cos \varphi(t)} \tag{8.13}$$

For a cosine oscillation with angular frequency ω_0, we can choose $a(t) = 1$ and $\varphi(t) = \omega_0 t$. For a sine wave, we can choose $a(t) = 1$ and $\varphi(t) = \omega_0 t - \pi/2$. However, this choice is not unique. For example, $a(t) = \cos \omega_0 t$ and $\varphi(t) = 0$ also produces the cosine wave. An extra requirement can be put on $a(t)$ that it is the most lowpass (slowest changing) of the possible functions satisfying Equation 8.13. This introduces uniqueness of the first of the afore-mentioned choices for the cosine and the sine waves.

This discussion suggests a definition of an *instantaneous angular frequency* by $\dot{\varphi}$. For the cosine and sine waves, we obtain $\dot{\varphi} = \omega_0$. $\dot{\varphi}$ has a close connection to the *time interval histogram* (TIH) to be discussed in Section 8.6B. For this, the distance between adjacent zero crossings (t_{k-1} and t_k) of the signal is used to produce a frequency estimate. Sainz, et al. have used a *phase-locked* loop technique to analyze the Doppler signal.[2] This produces an approximate estimate of $\dot{\varphi}$ if the loop is made fast. The zero-crossing counter which gives the average number of zero crossings per unit time has some resemblance to the TIH. This is discussed in Section 8.6.

B. Which Frequency Definition is Relevant?

Four frequency concepts have been introduced in the previous section:

1) the fundamental frequency of a strictly periodic signal;
2) the zero-crossing frequency for a semiperiodic signal;
3) the Fourier frequency; and
4) the instantaneous frequency.

Which frequency definition applies to the Doppler signal? As discussed, the second definition has meaning for a single scatterer, while the third and fourth have meaning for a composite signal from many scatterers, as from blood.

In answering this question, we first emphasize that our goal is to extract the maximum amount of information about the blood velocity from the signal. It can be shown that all information is contained in the signal *power spectrum*.[3] This can be defined as

$$G_x(\omega) = \lim_{T \to \infty} \frac{1}{T} E\{|X_T(\omega)|^2\} \tag{8.14}$$

where $X_T(\omega)$ is the Fourier transform of $x(t)$ over a time interval of length, T.[4] $E\{\ \}$ denotes averaging over an infinite number of blood flow systems that are identical except that the individual positions of the scatterers have a random variation from system to system. This is termed *ensemble averaging*.

From the physical viewpoint, we can interpret that

$$G_x(\omega)\, d\omega = \begin{cases} \textbf{the average amount of power of the signal} \\ \textbf{in the angular frequency interval } (\omega,\ \omega + d\omega) \end{cases}$$

Equation 8.14 is a purely mathematical definition of the power spectrum and cannot be used for computation. In the practical situation we know $x(t)$ for a time interval of length, T. We can then form an estimate of G_x by

$$\tilde{G}_x(\omega) = \frac{1}{T}|X_T(\omega)|^2 \tag{8.15}$$

This estimate will contain errors as discussed in Section 3.4B.

The conclusion we can draw is that the Fourier frequency is the relevant frequency to be used for Doppler signal analysis. The adequacy of the other frequency definitions to give information about the blood velocity can then be examined by analyzing how they relate to the signal power spectrum. As will be discussed in Section 8.6, the instantaneous frequency or TIH does not produce the detailed form of the power spectrum and, therefore, does not give as much information as Fourier analysis. In particular, it does not reveal the maximum velocity which is of special clinical importance. The same is true for the phase-locked loop analysis.

8.3 SPECTRUM OF DOPPLER SIGNAL FROM BLOOD

In Sections 3.4 and 3.6 we have discussed the relationship between the velocity profile and the signal power spectrum. A mathematical description of the Doppler signal is presented here, and we describe how the Doppler information can be extracted by quadrature demodulation. How to resolve the direction of velocities from the Doppler signal is also discussed. The complex Doppler signal is introduced as a convenient notation which takes care of the directionality.

A. Model of Composite Doppler Signal

As described in the previous section, the Doppler signal is a sum of bursts of oscillations with random position in time and different Doppler shifts in frequency. The return signal is, therefore, a truly random process. Since the signal is Gaussian, all information is contained in its power spectrum.[3]

It is easiest to model the received rf signal for the continuous wave Doppler instrument. For this we can write

$$u(t) = a(t) \cos \{\omega_0 t + \varphi(t)\} \tag{8.16}$$

where ω_0 is the angular frequency of the transmitted ultrasound. The equation describes an oscillation at rf frequencies with slowly varying amplitude, $a(t)$, and phase modulation, $\varphi(t)$. These contain the Doppler information and have a band width of the order of kHz. For the pulsed wave instrument, the description of the received signal is more complex.[3] Range resolution is obtained by sampling the return echo a certain time delay after the pulse transmission. By this, the Doppler signal from the range cell is reconstructed as if it were obtained with a CW instrument, provided the condition of the sampling theorem in Equation 3.7 is met. To simplify the basic ideas, we therefore proceed with Equation 8.16. It can be rewritten as

$$u(t) = x(t) \cos\omega_0 t - y(t) \sin\omega_0 t \tag{8.17}$$

where

$$x(t) = a(t) \cos \varphi(t)$$
$$y(t) = a(t) \sin \varphi(t)$$

(8.18)

These are called the *quadrature components* of the Doppler signal.

A typical power spectrum of u(t) is shown in Figure 8.3. The spectrum broadening of the received signal around ω_0 is determined by the Doppler shifts of the various backscattered bursts and the transit time effect discussed in Section 8.2A. If we neglect the transit time effect ($T_t \to \infty$), the signal with a single angular Doppler shift, ω_d, is

$$u(t) = \cos(\omega_o + \omega_d)t = \cos\omega_d t \cos\omega_o t - \sin\omega_d \sin\omega_o t$$
$$x(t) = \cos\omega_d t$$
$$y(t) = \sin\omega_d t$$

(8.19)

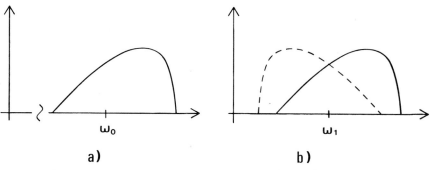

a)   b)

Fig. 8–3.   Received Doppler spectrum centered around ω_0 and ω_1.

B.   Demodulation; Offset Spectrum

In general, we can obtain x(t) from u(t) by multiplying with $2\cos\omega_0 t$ and low-pass filtering the product. Similarly, we obtain y(t) by multiplying u(t) with $-2\sin\omega_0 t$ followed by low-pass filtering. From Equation 8.17 we obtain

$$2u(t)\cos\omega_o t = x(t)[1 + \cos2\omega_o t] - y(t)\sin2\omega_o t$$

(8.20)

Upon low-pass filtering, the components with angular frequency $2\omega_0$ disappear and x(t) is extracted. A block diagram for the demodulation is shown in Figure 8.4a. For a PW instrument, x(t) and y(t) from a certain range cell

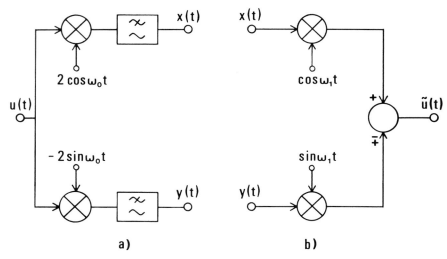

Fig. 8–4. a) Quadrature demodulation. b) Generation of offset Doppler spectrum around ω_1.

are obtained after sampling and low-pass filtering of the demodulated rf signal.

$x(t)$ and $y(t)$ contain all information in the signal. Since $\cos\omega_0 t$ and $\sin\omega_0 t$ are known signals, we can regenerate $u(t)$ from $x(t)$ and $y(t)$ using Equation 8.17. In fact, we can regenerate the same spectrum centered around an arbitrary angular frequency, ω_1, using the following formula

$$\tilde{u}(t) = x(t)\cos\omega_1 t \mp y(t)\sin\omega_1 t \tag{8.21}$$

If the $+$ sign in Equation 8.21 is used, the spectrum is inverted around ω_1, as indicated in Figure 8.3b.

C. Complex Envelope; Directional Information

To simplify the mathematical analysis, we can define a *complex envelope* of the rf signal as

$$\hat{x}(t) = x(t) + iy(t) \tag{8.22}$$

where $i = \sqrt{-1}$ is the imaginary unit. As will be evident in the following discussion, this is just a convenient way to handle all Doppler information, both $x(t)$ and $y(t)$, in one notation. By this means, Equations 8.16 and 8.17 can be rewritten as

$$u(t) = \text{Re}\,\{\hat{x}(t)\,e^{i\,\omega_0 t}\} \tag{8.23}$$

The complex signal

$$e(t) = \hat{x}(t)\,e^{i\omega_0 t} \qquad\qquad (8.24)$$

is termed the *analytic signal* of u (t) and has positive frequency components only (complex Fourier spectrum, see Section 8.2A).

The effect of the demodulation in Figure 8.4a is to move the positive frequency components, ω_0, downward and the negative frequency components, ω_0, upward along the angular frequency axis. This is illustrated in Figure 8.5. The rf signal contains both positive and negative Doppler shifts

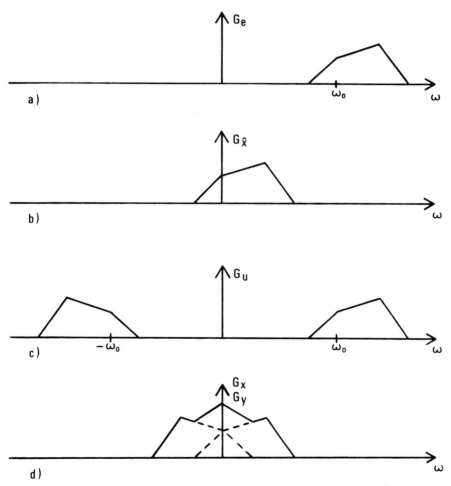

Fig. 8–5. The translation of the frequency spectrum in the demodulation. Power spectrum of analytic signal (a), complex envelope (b), real rf signal (c), and quadrature components (d).

around ω_0. We note that since u (t) is real, its power spectrum is symmetric around $\omega = 0$. This is evident from Equation 8.14 and the discussion following Equation 8.10. The power spectrum of e (t) has positive-frequency components only, as stated previously, and the spectrum of $\hat{x}$ (t) is asymmetric around $\omega = 0$ since $\hat{x}$ (t) is a complex signal.

The spectrum of the complex envelope takes care of the directional information. If we look at the spectrum of the quadrature components separately, however, the positive and negative Doppler shifts in u (t) become mixed up as the frequency components for $\omega < 0$ are moved $+\omega_0$ while the frequency components for $\omega > 0$ are moved $-\omega_0$. However, there is a special cross correlation between x and y; therefore, when we form the complex envelope $\hat{x} = x + iy$, the directional information is restored.

This is perhaps more easily understood if we look at the complex envelope $\hat{x}$ (t) as a phasor. For positive Doppler shifts, it rotates clockwise. This is seen from Equation 8.19, which gives for a single component

$$\hat{x}\,(t) = \cos\omega_d t + i\,\sin\omega_d t = e^{i\omega_d t} \qquad (8.25)$$

Thus, $\omega_d > 0$, x (t) is 90° in front of y (t), whereas for $\omega_d < 0$, y (t) is 90° in front of x (t). This concept is illustrated in Figure 8.6.

There are two ways to take care of the complete directional spectrum: 1) to use the complex Fourier transform on $\hat{x}$ (t), and 2) to generate a real signal with an offset spectrum as shown in Equation 8.21 and Figure 8.3. The property that the power spectrum of a complex signal can be asymmetric around $\omega = 0$ can be used to measure Doppler shifts higher than the Nyquist

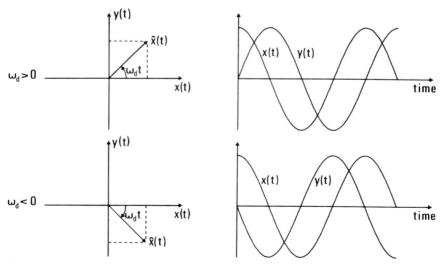

Fig. 8–6. Quadrature components and phasor for complex envelope for single-frequency Doppler signal. Upper panel shows $\omega_d > 0$ while lower panel shows $\omega_d < 0$. Note the relative phase-lag between x(t) and y (t).

rate for the pulsed Doppler instrument, as discussed in Sections 3.6 and 8.4C.

8.4 FOURIER ANALYSIS[1,5,6]

From Sections 8.2B and 8.3, it is clear that the computation of the Fourier spectrum is important in the analysis of Doppler signals. In the practical situation, we have a finite time sample of the Doppler signal. Therefore, it is the finite time Fourier transform, i.e., integration over a finite interval and not from $-\infty$ to ∞, which is important. In the following section we discuss the properties of the finite time transform and the use of a bank of band-pass filters to obtain it. The discrete Fourier transform (DFT) is another technique for obtaining the finite time transform, which has compact electronic implementations, such as the chirp-z transform and the fast Fourier transform. The DFT works on samples of the signal. Therefore, we briefly discuss the spectrum of sampled signals to give a better background on the sampling theorem and the limit on the range velocity product discussed in Sections 3.3B and 3.6. How the limit on the range velocity product can be increased by using complex spectral analysis is also indicated.

A. The Fourier Transform as a Filter; Windowing

The finite-time Fourier transform is obtained if we reduce the integration in Equation 8.6 to a finite time interval. Assume that we calculate the finite-time Fourier transform of $\cos \omega t$ at w. The Fourier transform is then a function of w, $X(w)$. If we keep w fixed and vary ω, a function $H_w(\omega) = X(w)$ is obtained. The amplidute $|H_w|$ is illustrated in Figure 8.7a. It has the form of a band-pass filter centered at w. The band width of the filter is

$$\triangle \omega = \frac{2\pi}{T} \tag{8.26}$$

where T is the length of the time interval for which the integration in the Fourier transform is performed.

The effect of finite time integration in the Fourier transform is automatically obtained if we multiply the signal $x(t)$ by a rectangular *time window,* $w_R(t)$, which is equal to unity in the interval in which we perform integration, and equal to zero outside it. This window is inserted in Figure 8.1a. The signal $x(t)$ inside the time window is called the *data sample.* The band width of the filter is therefore inversely proportional to the length of the data sample, T.

The side lobes in Figure 8.7a are also a notable property of this filter. The ratio of the amplitude of the nearest side lobe to the main lobe is

$$\alpha_R = .21 \qquad \sim - 13.4 \text{ dB} \tag{8.27}$$

where the subscript R denotes rectangular window.

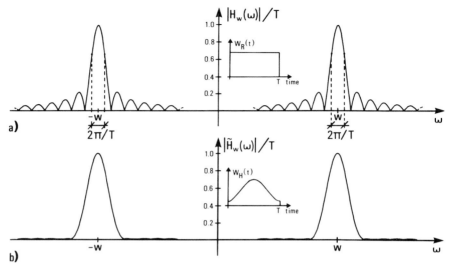

Fig. 8–7.   The Fourier transform as a filter. a) Unwindowed or equivalently rectangular window. b) Hamming window is used. The time windows are inserted.

Window functions other than the rectangular are mostly used to obtain a better response of the filter. A commonly used function is the Hamming window, $w_H(t)$, which is inserted in Figure 8.7b. The filter obtained using this window and the Fourier transform is also illustrated in Figure 8.7b. The side lobe ripple has been reduced to

$$\alpha_H = .0074 \qquad \sim -42.7 \text{ dB} \qquad\qquad (8.28)$$

The width of the main lobe of the Hamming window is twice that of the rectangular window.

The band width of the filter is thus increased at the same time as the side lobe level is decreased. This windowing is desirable in several situations. One is to reduce the uncertainty in the amplitude of a power spectrum estimate,[1,7] which is discussed in the next section. Another is to separate weak frequency components from strong frequency components in a composite signal. In this situation, although the rectangular window produces a narrower main lobe than the Hamming window, the latter has much better attenuation of frequencies outside the main lobe.

This concept is important in ultrasonic Doppler blood velocity measurements. Here we have strong reflections from vessel walls and valve cusps at low Doppler shifts, whereas the scattering from blood which has higher Doppler shifts is weaker. Although the low-frequency components are attenuated with high-pass filters, there are still remnants of these components in the signal that passes through the high-pass filter. If windowing is not used in the calculation of the Fourier transform, the signals from tissue can corroborate the signal from blood in the transform.

B.   The Use of a Band-Pass Filter to Obtain the Fourier Transform

The previous section explains how the finite-time Fourier transform can be viewed as a band-pass filter. In the same way, a band-pass filter can be used to obtain an approximation to the finite-time Fourier transform. A typical frequency response of a band-pass filter is shown in Figure 8.8. The output of the filter from a wide-band signal input is an oscillation with a slowly varying amplitude and inverse period angular frequency of ω. The amplitude has a partly random variation with an approximate "period" of

$$T = \frac{2\pi}{\triangle\omega} \tag{8.29}$$

This is an approximate measure for the rise time of the filter. That is, if we suddenly switch the input of the filter to a sinusoidal oscillation of angular frequency, w, the amplitude of the output rises slowly to the stationary value. The time necessary to obtain the stationary value of the amplitude is approximately given by Equation 8.29.

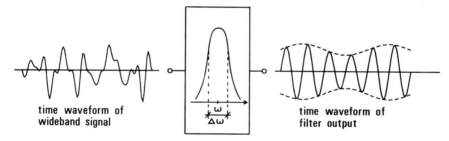

time waveform of
wideband signal

time waveform of
filter output

Fig. 8–8.   Band-pass filtering of a wideband signal.

The amplitude at the filter output is approximately the amplitude of the finite-time Fourier transform at w over a time interval, T. The approximation occurs since the filter frequency response is not identical to that in Figure 8.7a obtained with the Fourier transform. By using a bank of band-pass filters, we can then obtain an approximation to the signal Fourier transform at discrete frequency points, which is illustrated in Figure 8.9.

Since we are interested in the power spectrum (see Section 8.1B), we should square the filter output and perform low-pass filtering, as illustrated in Figure 8.10.

The oscillations in the filter output amplitude occur since the input is a random signal. They are the cause for the inaccuracy of the power spectrum estimate in finite time estimation. This is discussed in Sections 3.4B and 8.2B.

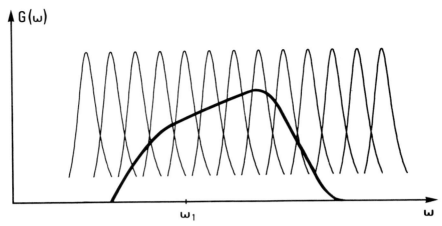

Fig. 8–9. Estimation of the Fourier transform at discrete points using a bank of band-pass filters.

The "period" of the amplitude variations is given by Equation 8.29. It is then evident that if the frequency accuracy, $\triangle\omega$, is kept constant and low-pass filtering of the square of the filter output is performed, the uncertainty in the power spectrum estimate is reduced.

The basic reason that the inaccuracy can be reduced is that the estimation time is increased, while the frequency accuracy is kept constant. The same can be obtained with the Fourier transform if we first calculate it for a long time, T, and produce the estimate

$$\hat{G}_x(\omega) = \frac{1}{T} \left| X_T(\omega) \right|^2 \qquad (8.30)$$

Then we can create a new estimate $\hat{G}_x(\omega)$ from $\hat{G}_x(\omega)$ by averaging $\hat{G}_x$ over neighboring frequencies.[1,7] This is illustrated in Figure 8.10b. The frequency averaging can be performed by convolution with a band-pass frequency window as illustrated in the figure. This is similar to multiplying with a window in the time domain. In fact, an often-used frequency window, W, is the Fourier transform of the Hamming window, $w_H(t)$.

If the frequency accuracy is inversely proportional to the analyzing time (see Equation 8.26), the uncertainty in the power spectrum estimate is independent of the analyzing time. For a band-pass filter, this is seen as a constant variation in the filter output amplitude, the period of the variation increasing as $\triangle\omega$ decreases (see Equation 8.29).

One might wonder why the uncertainty in the amplitude is not decreased in this case, since the amount of information increases with the length of the data sample. The reason is that we simultaneously narrow the band width of the filter so that the amount of information within the band-pass filter is kept constant.

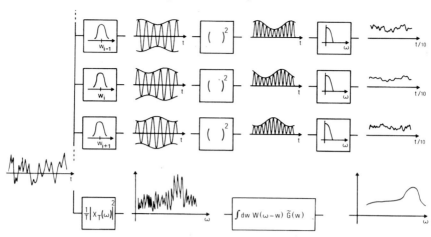

Fig. 8–10. Reduction of amplitude uncertainty in power spectrum estimate by low-pass filtering of band-pass output (a) and averaging in the frequency domain (b).

C.   Sampled Signals[5,6]

A sampled signal is a set of short pulses with height equal to the amplitude of the unsampled signal, as illustrated in Figure 8.11. The sampling can be performed by a switch which connects for a short interval at each sampling point in time.

Sampled signals have special importance in ultrasonic blood velocity measurements since, in the pulsed instrument, only samples of the Doppler

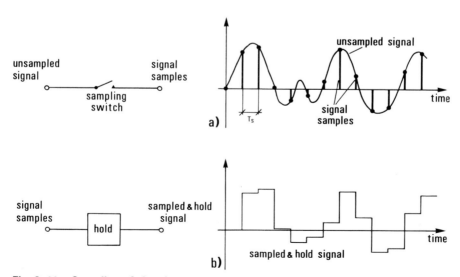

Fig. 8–11.   Sampling of signals.

signal are obtained. In addition, as discussed in the next section, some interesting spectrum analyzers work on sampled signals.

The distance in time between the samples is T_s. The sampling frequency, f_s, then becomes

$$f_s = \frac{1}{T_s} \tag{8.31}$$

Often the sampled signal is fed through a hold element which holds the value of the sample until the next sampling occurs. Then the hold element changes to the new sample value. This is illustrated in the lower panel of Figure 8.11.

The spectrum of a sampled signal is illustrated in Figure 8.12. The original signal has a low-pass spectrum. After sampling, this is repeated around $k\omega_s$, where $\omega_s = 2\pi f_s$ is the angular sampling frequency. If we are using a hold element, the amplitude of the repeated spectra decreases with $|\omega|$ because the hold function reduces the high frequency content in the signal, as shown in Figure 8.11b.

As illustrated in Figure 8.12b, if the sampled signal is passed through a low-pass filter with band width $\omega_s/2$, all the higher-order repeated spectra are rejected. The original signal spectrum and thereby the original signal are then restored.

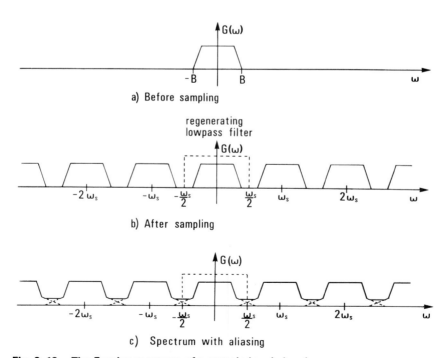

a) Before sampling

b) After sampling

c) Spectrum with aliasing

Fig. 8–12. The Fourier spectrum of a sampled real signal.

The criterion for this to occur is that the original signal has no frequency components greater than $\omega_s/2$. This is the *Shannon sampling theorem,* and $\omega_s/2$ is called the angular *Nyquist frequency.*

The spectrum in Figure 8.12 is symmetric around zero which means that the signal is real. If B is the signal band width, the requirement in the Shannon sampling theorem for errorless reconstruction of *real* signals is

$$\mathbf{B} < \frac{\mathbf{f_s}}{2} \tag{8.32}$$

If $B > f_s/2$, as indicated by the stippling in Figure 8.12c, frequency components from the bands centered around $\pm f_s$ fall into the regenerating filter band from $-f_s/2$ to $f_s/2$. This phenomenon is termed *aliasing.* When it occurs, it is not possible to regenerate the original signal from the samples as shown in Figure 8.12c. This phenomenon sets a limit on the maximum Doppler shift that can be measured with a pulsed Doppler instrument, as discussed in Sections 3.3 and 3.6.

If the signal is complex, the spectrum may not be symmetric around $\omega = 0$ as illustrated in Figure 8.13. Here we are able to regenerate the original signal even if

$$\omega_{max} > \frac{\omega_s}{2}$$

provided

$$\omega_{max} - \omega_{min} < \omega_s \tag{8.33}$$

Thus, if we have a complex representation of the Doppler signal, as described in Section 8.3C, we are able to analyze Doppler shifts higher than the Nyquist frequency. This phenomenon is discussed in Section 3.6. In addition, if ω_{max} is increased as in Figure 8.13c, the excess positive frequencies will, due to aliasing, be found as negative frequencies in the regenerating filter. The same phenomenon is demonstrated in Figures 3.19, 3.21, and 3.22.

D. The Discrete Fourier Transform (DFT)[5,6]

Section 8.4B describes how an approximation to the amplitude of the Fourier transform in a set of discrete points can be obtained with a bank of band-pass filters. The Fourier transform can also be obtained, under certain conditions, in a set of discrete frequency points using what is called the discrete Fourier transform:

$$\mathbf{X_k} = \sum_{n=0}^{N-1} \mathbf{x_n}\, e^{-i\frac{2\pi}{N}kn} \tag{8.34}$$

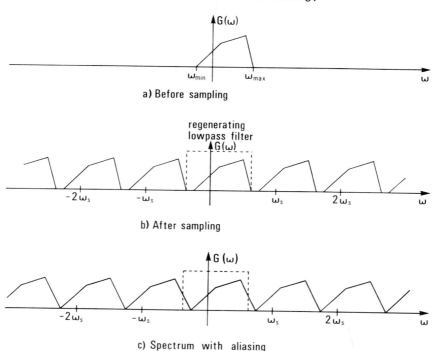

a) Before sampling

b) After sampling

c) Spectrum with aliasing

Fig. 8–13.   The Fourier spectrum of a sampled complex signal.

x_n, n = 0, 1, ---, and N−1 represent N samples of the time waveform, x (t). The sampling occurs at fixed intervals of length, T_s. A set of N complex frequency components (X_k, k = 0, 1, ---, and N − 1) is then produced. The angular frequency corresponding to frequency component number k is

$$\omega_k = \frac{2\pi}{T} k \qquad\qquad (8.35)$$

where T = NT_s is the analyzing time as in the previous sections. ω_1 is called the *fundamental angular frequency,* and the other frequency components are *harmonics* of this frequency component. The mapping in Equation 8.34 can be inverted:

$$x_n = \frac{1}{N} \sum_{k=0}^{N-1} X_k \, e^{i\frac{2\pi}{N}kn} \qquad\qquad (8.36)$$

Thus, the time and the frequency samples are related through a DFT pair.
  The DFT produces samples of the Fourier transform of the *sampled signal.* This is illustrated in Figure 8.14 for both a real and a complex signal whose spectra are shown in Figures 8.12 and 8.13. Since the spectrum of a sampled

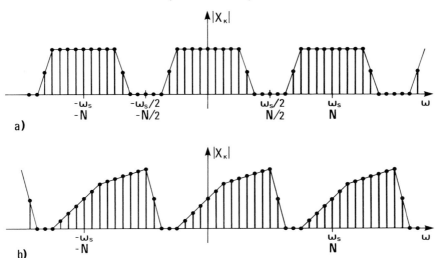

Fig. 8–14. DFT of real signal with spectrum in Figure 8-12(a) and complex signal with spectrum in Figure 8-13(b).

signal is repeated around harmonics of the sampling frequency, this periodicity also occurs for the DFT and the phenomenon of *aliasing* also applies.

The DFT of a cosine wave (equivalently sine wave) is particularly interesting. The continuous Fourier transform of a cosine wave is shown in Figure 8.2. If the analyzing interval, T, is an integer number of signal periods, the DFT samplings of the spectrum occur in the center of the main lobe, and then in all the zeros of X (ω). This is illustrated in Figure 8.15a. The DFT is then zero for all ks except for the k that satisfies

$$\omega = \frac{2\pi}{T}k \qquad (8.37)$$

where ω is the angular frequency of the cosine wave. If no k exists, so that Equation 8.37 is satisfied, several X_ks will be different from zero, as illustrated in Figure 8.15b.

Often, spectrum analyzers that compute the DFT have a hold element at the output so that the output resembles the stippled curves in Figure 8.15.

It is sometimes desirable that the DFT produce a sampling of the continuous spectrum that is denser than the one in Figure 8.15. This can be achieved if the length of the signal to be analyzed is T_0. The data sample is then extended by filling in with zeros as shown in Figure 8.16. The actual analyzing time is then T so that the distance between the frequency samples in the DFT is

$$\triangle\omega = \frac{2\pi}{T} \qquad (8.38)$$

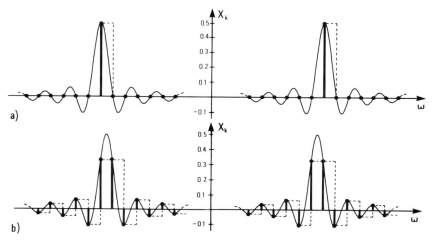

Fig. 8–15. DFT of a cosine wave. The analyzing interval is an integer number of wave periods (a) and a noninteger number of wave periods (b).

while the distance between the zeros in the continuous Fourier transform is

$$\triangle\omega_0 = \frac{2\pi}{T_o} \tag{8.39}$$

E.   Accuracy of Frequency Determination

The distance between the frequency samples in the DFT is

$$\triangle f = \frac{1}{T} \tag{8.40}$$

where $T = NT_s$ is the analyzing time. This gives $\triangle f = f_s/N$. The distance between samples is equal to the width of the main lobe of a sine wave analyzed over the same period, as discussed in Section 8.2A. Thus, for a signal that is composed for several sine waves, the accuracy by which we can determine the zero-crossing frequency of the different components is given by Equation 8.40.

Equation 8.40 is sometimes called the uncertainty relation of the Fourier transform. It is similar to the uncertainty relation in quantum mechanics with one basic difference: In quantum mechanics the functions involved are interpreted as probabilities. The similarity is therefore purely mathematical and is a property of the Fourier transform.

As discussed in Section 8.2A, the inaccuracy in determining the zero-crossing frequency from the Fourier transform arises from noise in the signal. The interpretation of Equation 8.40 as an accuracy in our case is therefore loose.

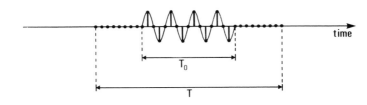

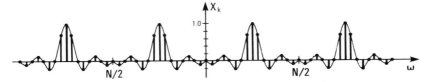

Fig. 8–16. **Decreasing the sampling interval along the frequency axis by extending the data sample with zeros.**

8.5 TECHNIQUES OF COMPUTING THE DFT

The computation of the DFT from Equation 8.34 can be tedious in the practical situation. However, there are two special methods of computation, the chirp-z transform and the fast Fourier transform (FFT), that are practical for Doppler signal analysis. These are described in this section.

A. Chirp-Z Transform

The detailed computation of the DFT can be changed by using the following substitution in the exponential in Equation 8.34:

$$2kn = k^2 + n^2 - (k-n)^2 \tag{8.41}$$

For the power spectrum, we are interested in the square of the Fourier transform, which also simplifies the computation. In Equation 8.34 it is assumed that we use the same set of samples to calculate all frequency components. If we have a stationary signal (i.e., velocity profile time stationary), we can shift the set of samples one step for each k. This is called the *sliding transform* and simplifies the calculations further. The computation can then be split into a premultiplication of $\hat{x}_n$ with a linear frequency chirp. Convolution is then performed with filters whose impulse responses are frequency chirps. A block diagram of the chirp-z computation is shown in Figure 8.17. With the sliding transform, the windowing discussed in Section 8.4A can be incorporated in the convolution filters as described by Brodersen, et al.[8]

The convolution filters can be implemented using charge transfer devices. This gives a simple and elegant hardware realization for the analyzer with accuracy and dynamic range which are suitable for Doppler signal analysis.

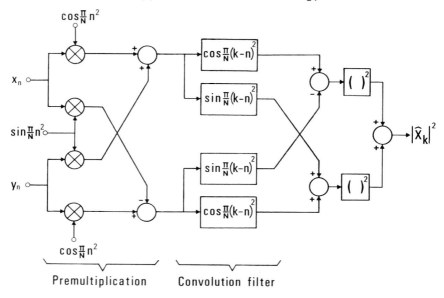

Fig. 8–17. Block diagram of chirp-z transform for power spectrum estimation.

A dynamic range of 60 dB has been obtained in our laboratory, using the R5602 chirp filter. To obtain a comparable dynamic range with the FFT algorithm discussed in the next section, 10 bits are necessary in the digitization of the analogue input wave form.

The analyzer works on discrete time samples of the signal and produces a set of discrete frequency samples. The distance between the frequency points is $\Delta f = 1/T$ from Equation 8.40, and the total frequency range of the analyzer is $N\Delta f$ where N is the number of time (and frequency) samples.

B. Fast Fourier Transform FFT[6]

The FFT algorithm is a special way to calculate the DFT so that the number of multiplications is minimized. The algorithm can be conveniently implemented in a digital computer or microprocessor system. Special hardwired digital systems for computation of the FFT also exist.

The complex DFT as given in Equation 8.34 requires $(N-1)^2$ complex multiplications and $N(N-1)$ complex additions. Thus, for reasonably large values of N, direct calculations of the DFT require a large amount of computation. However, by taking into account the periodicity of the complex exponential function, we can reduce the number of multiplications. In this process the original N-point sequence is broken into two shorter sequences, the DFTs of which can be combined to give the DFT of the original N-point sequence. The two sequences are then broken into four new ones and so on until we have subsequences consisting of two samples only. For this to occur, N must be of the form 2^i. These two samples are combined in a *butterfly* operation. If the two samples are A and B, the outputs of the operation are

$$\mathbf{X} = \mathbf{A} + \mathbf{W}^k\,\mathbf{B}$$
$$\mathbf{Y} = \mathbf{A} - \mathbf{W}^k\,\mathbf{B}$$

(8.42)

where we have defined

$$\mathbf{W}^k = \mathbf{e}^{-i\frac{2\pi}{N}k}$$

(8.43)

The butterfly operation is illustrated in Figure 8.18. The whole FFT algorithm is then composed of a set of butterfly operations which are illustrated for an eight-point FFT in Figure 8.19.

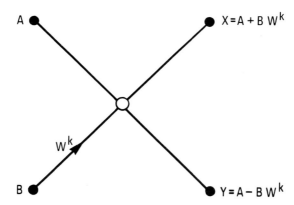

Fig. 8–18. Butterfly operation.

The FFT is implemented digitally, and the accuracy and dynamic range are determined by how many bits are used in the digitization of the analogue signals. For example, an eight-bit FFT has a dynamic range of 38 dB for the minimum and maximum rms value of a Gaussian signal that can be analyzed. The FFTs implemented for Doppler signal analysis are usually eight-bit, which give a dynamic range that is somewhat inferior to what can be obtained by the chirp-z transform and CTD devices, discussed in the previous section.

8.6 SIMPLIFIED FORMS OF SPECTRAL ANALYSIS

In Section 8.3 it is stated that the Doppler signal can be modeled by a Gaussian random process. From this, several interesting properties of the signal can be deduced. These properties clarify some simplified methods of spectrum analysis that have been used.

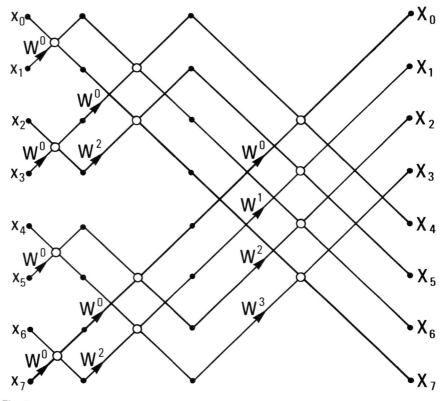

Fig. 8–19.   Calculation flow diagram of eight-point FFT algorithm.

A.   Instantaneous and Mean Frequency

The complex envelope in Equation 8.22 can be rewritten as

$$\hat{x}(t) = a(t)\,e^{i\varphi(t)}$$

$$a(t) = \sqrt{x^2(t) + y^2(t)} \tag{8.44}$$

$$\varphi(t) = \tan^{-1}\left\{\frac{y(t)}{x(t)}\right\}$$

With this notation, we can express the quadrature components of the Doppler signal (See Equation 8.22) as

$$x(t) = \text{Re}\left\{\hat{x}(t)\right\} = a(t)\cos\varphi(t) \quad \text{a)}$$

$$y(t) = \text{Im}\left\{\hat{x}(t)\right\} = a(t)\sin\varphi(t) \quad \text{b)} \tag{8.45}$$

The instantaneous angular Doppler frequency is then defined as the derivative of the phase φ

$$\dot{\varphi}(t) = \frac{d\varphi}{dt} \tag{8.46}$$

$\dot{\varphi}(t)$ is a function of time. If the velocity profile is stationary and we perform averaging of $\dot{\varphi}$, we obtain the mean angular frequency, $\overline{\omega}$, of the spectrum.[9] $\overline{\omega}$ can be obtained from the spectrum by integration:

$$\overline{\omega} = \frac{\int\limits_{-\infty}^{\infty} d\omega \, \omega \, G_{\hat{x}}(\omega)}{\int\limits_{-\infty}^{\infty} d\omega \, G_{\hat{x}}(\omega)} \tag{8.47}$$

This is called the *first moment* of the spectrum. A more detailed discussion of both the mean and the instantaneous frequencies of the Doppler signal is given by Angelsen.[9]

Although $\dot{\varphi}$ has the appeal of being a frequency, as discussed in Section 8.2, its relation to the Fourier spectrum is fairly complex. If we observe the density distribution for the relative time $\dot{\varphi}$ spends in intervals ($\dot{\varphi}$, $\dot{\varphi} + d\dot{\varphi}$), a bell-shaped curve centered around $\overline{\omega}$ is found. This function is called the first-order probability density for $\dot{\varphi}$ and is shown in Figure 8.20. The density is completely determined by $\overline{\omega}$ and $\overline{\omega^2}$:

$$\overline{\omega^2} = \frac{\int\limits_{-\infty}^{\infty} d\omega \, \omega^2 \, G_{\hat{x}}(\omega)}{\int\limits_{-\infty}^{\infty} d\omega \, G_{\hat{x}}(\omega)} \tag{8.48}$$

This is the *second moment* of the spectrum. The *root mean square* (rms) frequency of the spectrum is defined as

$$\omega_{rms} = \sqrt{\overline{\omega^2}} \tag{8.49}$$

The rms spectral band width is defined as

$$B_{rms} = \sqrt{\overline{\Delta\omega^2}} = \frac{\int\limits_{-\infty}^{\infty} d\omega \, (\omega - \overline{\omega})^2 \, G_{\hat{x}}(\omega)}{\int\limits_{-\infty}^{\infty} d\omega \, G_{\hat{x}}(\omega)} \tag{8.50}$$

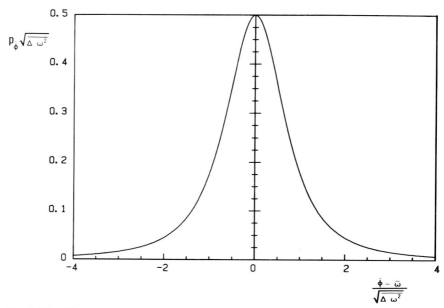

Fig. 8–20. First-order probability density for the instantaneous frequency.

which can be obtained from $\overline{\omega}$ and $\overline{\omega^2}$

$$\overline{\Delta\omega^2} = \overline{\omega^2} - \overline{\omega}^2 \qquad (8.51)$$

From the first-order probability density of $\dot{\varphi}$ it is then possible to obtain the mean frequency and the rms band width, but not the detailed form of the spectrum.

B. Time Interval Histogram (TIH)[10]

In this case, by the use of Equation 8.21, the Doppler signal is centered around so high a frequency ($\sim$50 kHz) that it becomes a narrow band. Most of the zero crossings of the signal are then determined by φ (t) in Equations 8.44 and 8.45. Let t_{k-1} and t_k denote two adjacent zero crossings of the Doppler signal. Then an approximation to $\dot{\varphi}$ can be obtained:

$$w_k = \frac{\pi}{t_k - t_{k-1}} \qquad (8.52)$$

For ordinary (not angular) frequency we obtain

$$v_k = \frac{w_k}{2\pi} = \frac{1}{2(t_k - t_{k-1})} \qquad (8.53)$$

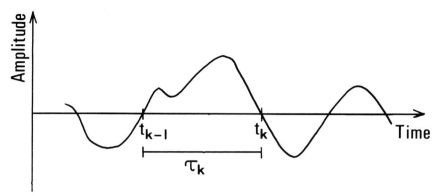

Frequency estimate: $v_k = \frac{1}{2\tau_k}$

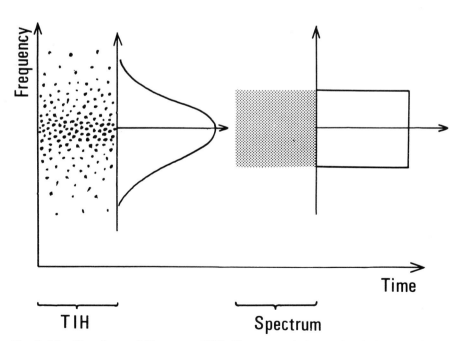

TIH   Spectrum

Fig. 8–21. Time interval histogram (TIH). Upper panel shows the derivation of the frequency estimate from the time waveform. The lower left panel shows the time-density plot of the TIH from a signal with a rectangular spectrum whose time-grey-scale plot is shown in the lower right panel.

A new estimate of the instantaneous frequency is then obtained for every zero crossing.

If the Doppler signal consists of a single frequency, i.e., a sine wave, v_k will give the exact frequency of the signal. When the signal spectrum widens, a scatter of the v_k·s around the mean frequency is obtained. This is illustrated in Figure 8.21. The upper panel illustrates how the frequency estimate is obtained from the time waveform of the signal. The lower left panel shows how the v_ks obtained for each pair of zero crossings can be plotted in a time-density diagram. The lower right panel shows a time-grey-scale plot of the power spectrum of the same signal (see Section 3.4B). The spectrum is supposed to have a square density as indicated to the right in the panel. This produces a bell-shaped TIH density as shown to the right in the lower left panel.

The darkness of the TIH scatter diagram is given by the first-order probability density of v.[11] For a narrow band signal, this is approximately equal to the probability density for $\dot{\varphi}$.[9] The TIH thus gives the mean frequency of the spectrum and the rms band width of the spectrum. It does not provide the detailed form of the spectrum, however, and spectra with different forms but with the same rms bandwith produce the same TIH.[11, 12]

C.   Maximum Frequency Estimation and Phase-Locked Loop

As discussed in Section 3.5A, there is no mathematical definition of the maximum frequency shift. A special estimator for a quasi maximum frequency is presented in the same section. Sainz, et al. have used a phase-locked loop technique to produce what they claim is the maximum frequency.[7] However, adequate results have not yet been proved with this technique. A fast loop should be expected to produce an approximation to the instantaneous frequency which does not give the maximum frequency.

D.   Zero-Crossing Counter

The zero-crossing counter averages the number of zero crossings per unit time and uses it as an estimate for the frequency. It can be shown that this estimate is equal to the rms (root mean square) frequency of the spectrum.[4] This frequency lies somewhere between the mean frequency and the maximum frequency of the spectrum as discussed in Section 3.5.

REFERENCES

1. Papoulis A.: Signal Analysis. New York, McGraw-Hill Book Co., 1977.
2. Sainz A., Roberts V.C., Pinardi G.: Phase-locked loop techniques applied to ultrasonic Doppler signal processing. Ultrasonics 1976; 3: 128-132.
3. Angelsen B.A.J.: A theoretical study of the scattering of ultrasound from blood. IEEE Trans. Biomed. Eng. 1980; BME-27: 61-67.
4. Papoulis A.: Probability, Random Variables and Stochastic Processes. New York, McGraw-Hill Book Co.,1965.
5. Harris F.J.: On the use of windows for harmonic analysis with the discrete Fourier transform. Proc. IEEE 1978; 66: 51-83.

6. Rabiner L.R., Gold B.: Theory and Application of Digital Signal Processing. Englewood Cliffs, N.J., Prentice-Hall, Inc., 1975.
7. Jenkins G.M., Watts D.G.: Spectral Analysis. London, Holden Day, 1969.
8. Brodersen R.W., Hewes C.R., Buss D.D.: A 500-stage CCD transversal filter for spectral analysis. IEEE Trans. Electron Dev. 1976; ED-23: 143-152.
9. Angelsen B.A.J.: Instantaneous frequency, mean frequency and variance of mean frequency esitmators for ultrasonic blood velocity Doppler signals. IEEE Trans. Biomed. Eng. 1981; 28: 733-741.
10. Baker D.W., Rubenstein G.A., Lorch G.S.: Pulsed Doppler endocardiography: Principles and applications. Am. J. Med. 1977; 63: 69-80.
11. Angelsen B.A.J.: Spectral estimation of a narrow-band Gaussian process from the distribution of the distance between adjacent zeros. IEEE Trans. Biomed Eng. 1980; BME-27: 108-110.
12. Burckhardt C.B.: Comparison between spectrum and time interval histogram of ultrasound Doppler signals. Ultrasound Med. Biol. 1981; 7: 79-82.

Appendix A

A1   CALCULATION OF VOLUMETRIC FLOW RATE FROM THE VELOCITY PROFILE

The velocity profile in an artery can be described as a function of the coordinates of the cross section:

$$\mathbf{v}(x,y) \tag{A1}$$

This is illustrated in Figure A1. We divide the cross section into areas ΔA which are so small that the velocity profile can be considered essentially constant across the area element. According to Equation 2.14, the volumetric flow through such an element is then

$$\Delta q_i \approx \Delta A\ \mathbf{v}(x_i,\ y_i) \tag{A2}$$

The volumetric flow rate through the whole cross section can be calculated as

$$q = \sum_{i=1}^{N} \Delta q_i \approx \sum_{i=1}^{N} \Delta A\ \mathbf{v}(x_i,\ y_i) \tag{A3}$$

The approximation arises because the velocity profile is not completely constant across ΔA. The smaller we make each area element ΔA, the better the approximation becomes. However, the number of elements increases in the inverse proportion and it becomes more tedious to calculate the sum in Equation A3. If we let $\Delta A \to O$, the sum changes to an integral and the approximation becomes exact. We thus obtain

$$q = \iint dA\ \mathbf{v}(x,\ y) \tag{A4}$$

Using Equation 2.15, we obtain for the space average velocity

$$\overline{\mathbf{v}} = \frac{1}{A}q = \frac{1}{A} \iint dA\ \mathbf{v}(x,\ y) \tag{A5}$$

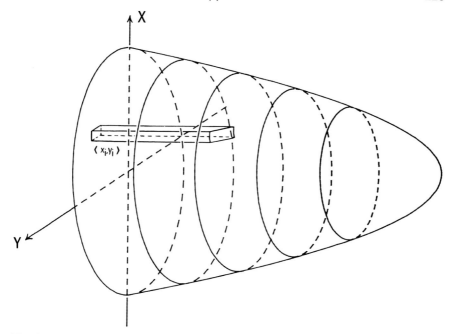

Fig. A1. Coordinates for velocity profile.

In the case of circular symmetry of the vessel and the profile, Equations A4 and A5 can be simplified. Assume that the velocity profile is of the form $v(r)$, where r is the distance from the axis as illustrated in Figure A1. The area of the infinitesimal ring in Figure A2 is

$$\mathbf{dA} = 2\pi \mathbf{r}\ \mathbf{dr} \tag{A6}$$

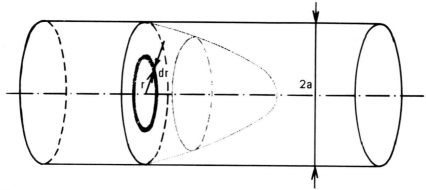

Fig. A2. Circular symmetric velocity profile.

and the volumetric flow can be calculated as

$$q = 2\pi \int_0^a dr\; r\; v(r) \tag{A7}$$

Actual flow profiles can often be approximated by the following formula:

$$v(r) = v_0\left[1 - \left(\frac{r}{a}\right)^n\right] \tag{A8}$$

$n = 2$ produces a parabolic profile and $n \to \infty$ represents a flat profile. Different profiles are shown in Figure A3. The volumetric flow is

$$q = 2\pi v_0 \int_0^a dr\; r\left[1 - \frac{r^n}{a^n}\right] \tag{A9}$$

$$= 2\pi v_0 \left|_0^a \frac{r^2}{2} - \frac{1}{n+2}\; \frac{r^{n+2}}{a^n}\right.$$

$$q = \frac{\pi a^2 v_0\; n}{n+2} \tag{A10}$$

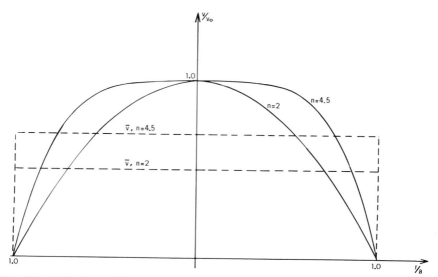

Fig. A3. Velocity profiles and mean velocity for $n = 2$ (parabolic) and $n = 4.5$ (accelerated).

The mean velocity in the artery is

$$\overline{v} = \frac{q}{\pi a^2} = v_0 \frac{n}{n+2} \tag{A11}$$

For the parabolic profile we obtain

$$\overline{v} = \frac{1}{2} v_0 \tag{A12}$$

$$q = \frac{1}{2} \pi a^2 v_0$$

That is, the mean velocity is half the maximum velocity in the artery. The accelerated profile in early systole can be approximately described by n = 4.5 which gives

$$\overline{v} = 0.7 \, v_0 \tag{A13}$$

In this case, if we use the maximum velocity to estimate cardiac stroke volume as discussed in Chapter 7, we should multiply the result by 0.7 to obtain correct results.

Appendix B

B1 OPTIMIZATION OF DOPPLER SYSTEM

For a Doppler system the important aspects in the optimization are

1) S/N ratio (signal-to-noise power ratio);
2) limit on the maximum measurable velocity; and
3) resolution.

The points are ranked according to importance in the clinical situation. Although it is not difficult to obtain a good signal-to-noise ratio in many patients, poor S/N ratio most often limits the applicability of a Doppler examination.

The backscattered power from a single scatterer is proportional to the ultrasonic frequency (f_0) in the fourth power,[1] i.e.,

$$\mathbf{S_s} \sim \mathbf{f_0}^4 \tag{B1}$$

where S_s denotes single scatterer signal power and $\sim$ denotes proportionality. However, in blood there is a distribution of scatterers, and the backscattered signal power is then proportional to the volume of the range cell.[1]

To be more clear, we should split the signal into one part carrying interesting information (S_i) and another part which is garbage (S_g). In a stenotic jet, for example, we are interested in the maximum velocity in the jet. The amount of blood moving with this velocity is limited to some region in space. If the range cell covers more than this region, the signal from this other part is garbage. Increasing the size of the range cell increases the signal power (S_i) from the maximum velocity region, only as long as the volume of blood moving with this velocity within the range cell increases. This is illustarted in Figure B1.

The longitudinal size (L) of the range cell is determined by the length of the transmitted pulse. The receiver band width (B) can be reduced when the

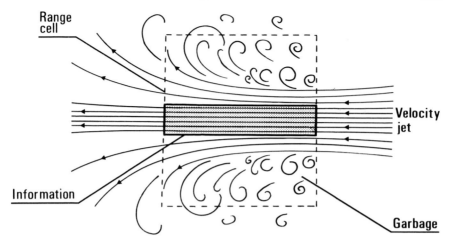

Fig. B1.   Origin of information carrying part of the signal and garbage.

pulse length is increased, thus reducing receiver noise power, $N \sim B$. For a fixed acoustic beam with diameter (D), the S/N ratio is then

$$\frac{S}{N} \sim f_0^4 \, \pi D^2 L^2 \qquad \text{(B2)}$$

$\pi D^2 L$ represents the volume of the range cell. *We thus see that good resolution and good S/N ratio are opposing requirements.* In many cases the S/N ratio is so poor that we must sacrifice resolution to increase the ratio. Noting the sound wavelength $\lambda = c/f_0$, we can rewrite Equation B2:

$$\frac{S}{N} \sim \left(\frac{D}{\lambda}\right)^2 \left(\frac{L}{\lambda}\right)^2 \qquad \text{(B3)}$$

If the size of the range cell is kept constant in terms of number of wavelengths, the S/N ratio is independent of the ultrasonic frequency.

We should remember that the signal in Equations B2 and B3 is composed of both information and garbage:

$$S = S_i + S_g \qquad \text{(B4)}$$

These statements are true for the information-carrying signal power only as long as S_i and S_g change in the same proportion when the size of the range cell is changed.

If the frequency is kept constant and we increase the size of the range cell, we reach some limit where S_i stops increasing since all blood-giving information-carrying signals are covered. However, the noise power is still $\sim B \sim L^{-1}$, i.e., in this case

$$\frac{S_i}{N} \sim L \tag{B5}$$

If we keep the size of the range cell constant in terms of wavelengths and vary the frequency, we have $B \sim f_0$. Thus, reducing f_0 always reduces $N \sim B$. If all the blood-giving information-carrying signals are covered by the range cell, we then have

$$\frac{S_i}{N} \sim f_0{}^3 \tag{B6}$$

Thus, decreasing the frequency when the range cell is kept constant in terms of wavelengths first leaves the S_i/N ratio unchanged (Equation B3). Then when interesting velocity inside the range cell stops increasing, the S_i/N ratio starts to fall off as $f_0{}^3$ (Equation B6).

The maximum velocity that can be measured at a depth (R) is inversely proportional to the ultrasonic frequency (see Figure 3.5). Thus, in order to measure high velocities, it is desirable to use as low an ultrasonic frequency as possible. Then to maintain (S_i/N) ratio, we need to increase the size of the range cell. However, as discussed in accordance with Equation B6, the decrease in frequency cannot be carried on indefinitely without decreasing the S_i/N ratio.

Practical considerations have then led to the choice of $f_0 = 2$ MHz. This gives a maximum measurable velocity of 1.7 m/s between 2 and 9 cm and 1.1 m/s between 9 and 12 cm. The resolution along the beam is set to approximately 7 mm, and a practical transducer size gives a beam diameter of approximately 7 mm. Thus, the diameter of the range cell is about 7 mm and its length is about 7 mm. These dimensions are not sharp since the beam has a slow decrease in intensity, as illustrated in Figure 3.1. The received pulse from a single scatterer also has a slow rise and decay due to band limitations in transducer and receiver. This makes the longitudinal resolution also only approximate.

Another reason for not having too small a range cell is the practical problem of locating disturbed flows. Since the heart structures are constantly moving, it is practical to let the size of the range cell be so large that the blood jet does not move out of it. In addition, a small range cell makes location of the disturbed flow more difficult.

B2 OPTIMIZATION OF AMPLITUDE IMAGING SYSTEM

For a pulse-echo amplitude imaging system, the critical points are

1) resolution and
2) penetration or S/N ratio.

The resolution is proportional to the frequency, whereas penetration is inversely proportional to the frequency. For cardiac measurements, one then ends up with an ultrasonic frequency of 2 to 3.5 MHz. The transmitted pulse has only a couple of oscillations, giving a longitudinal resolution of about 1 mm, in contrast to the 7 mm for the Doppler system. To obtain this, one backs the transducer with absorbing backing to widen the band width. This reduces the S/N ratio which is tolerable for an amplitude imaging system.

REFERENCES

1. Angelsen B.A.J.: A theoretical study of the scattering of ultrasound from Blood. IEEE Trans. Biomed. Eng. 1980; BME-27: 61-67.

Index

Numbers in *italics* indicate figures; numbers followed by a 't' indicate tables.

233